Publisher's Cataloging-In-Publication Data
(Prepared by The Donohue Group, Inc.)

Names: Anderson, J. Burton.
Title: Marijuana -- the wonder weed : everything you
    need to know and why it *must* be legalized / by:
    J. Burton Anderson, ChE, founder: The National
    Weed Legalization Fund.
Description: First edition rev. 1. | Green Valley,
    Arizona : Lions Pride Publishing, [2016]
Identifiers: ISBN 978-1-893257-84-9(paperback) |
    ISBN 978-1-893257-85-6 (Kindle) | ISBN 978-1-
    504354-88-7 (Google Play) |
    ISBN 978-1-893257-86-3 (ebook) | ISBN 978-1-
    893257-89-4 (pdf) | ISBN 978-1-893257-87-0
    (audiobook)
Subjects: LCSH: Marijuana. | Marijuana--Law and
    legislation--United States. | Marijuana--
    Therapeutic use. | Drug legalization--United
    States. | BISACSH: HEALTH & FITNESS / Alternative
    Therapies. | SOCIAL SCIENCE / Disease & Health
    Issues. | POLITICAL SCIENCE / Public
    Policy/Social Policy. | MEDICAL / Pain Medicine.
    | HISTORY / Social History.
Classification: LCC HV5822.M3 A54 2016 (print) | LCC
    HV5822.M3 (ebook) | DDC 362.29/5--dc23

MARIJUANA - THE WONDER WEED

EVERYTHING YOU NEED TO KNOW AND WHY IT *MUST* BE LEGALIZED

By: J. Burton Anderson, ChE
Founder: The National Weed Legalization Fund

Create Space Paperback – First Edition Rev. 1
ISBN #: 978-1-893257-84-9
Copyright © 2016
Lions Pride Publishing, Amado, Arizona
SAN: 299-7401
IBPA Member #126139

**Book Commissioned By Glenn E. Martin, CEO
WEED, Inc., Tucson, Arizona (Stock: BUDZ)
http://www.marijuana-farms.com**

i

DEDICATIONS

Dedicated to all of my fellow veterans. Have faith. Relief is just an election or two away.

To my beautiful wife of 32 years, Melanie, whose patience and understanding allows me the endless hours of researching and writing while she works a demanding 9 to 5 job and still manages to keep our gardens green and our household from falling apart!

To the late genius author and mentor Dan Poynter, who passed away in 2015. His guidance and instruction over the last four decades has inspired me to write many books on topics of importance. May he rest in peace.

And with special thanks to Glenn E. Martin, CEO of *WEED, Inc., Tucson, Arizona (Stock: BUDZ) for sharing his extensive knowledge of the marijuana industry, and for allowing me open access to his army of expert consultants.

*The author is a paid chemical engineering consultant, blogger and writer for WEED, Inc.

DISCLAIMERS

All material in this book is for <u>educational purposes</u> ONLY. Nothing in this book is meant to be medical or prescriptive advice in any way. This book contains information about illegal substances, with emphasis on marijuana and its derivatives. The author and publisher would like to emphasize that marijuana is, at this writing, federally illegal in the United States and its territories, and also throughout most of the countries on earth.

The possession, use, cultivation or sale of marijuana in any form can carry very heavy penalties. These penalties threaten the liberty and future livelihood of anyone convicted of these indiscretions. Even in states where federal law is bypassed and various levels of legality exist there is both strict local regulation AND the ever-present threat of federal intervention.

Every effort has been made to make this book as complete and accurate as possible. However, there may be mistakes in typography or content. The author and publisher do not warrant that the information contained in this book is fully complete or entirely correct and shall not be responsible for any errors or omissions.

This book is for information purposes only and does not impart legal, accounting, financial, investment or any other form of business advice to readers who must consult their own professional advisors before taking any action of any kind concerning any marijuana-related security or business.

We strongly recommend that you do your own research and confirmation of the information contained in this book . This

"could," "intends," "estimate," "anticipate," "plan," "predict" "probable," "potential," "possible," "should," "continue," and other words of similar meaning.

Actual results could differ materially from these forward-looking statements as a result of a number of risks. Given these risks and uncertainties, investors are cautioned not to place undue reliance on such forward-looking statements and no assurances can be given that such statements will be achieved.

Readers are advised to review SEC periodic reports: Forms 10-Q, 10-K, Form 8-K, insider reports, and Forms 3, 4, 5 Schedule 13-D. Lions Pride Publishing does not offer any such advice or analysis, and further urges you to consult your own independent tax, business, financial, legal and investment advisors. Investing in marijuana micro-cap and growth securities is highly speculative and carries and extremely high degree of risk. It is possible that an investor's investment may be reduced or lost entirely due to the highly speculative nature of the marijuana industry itself and the companies profiled.

IMPORTANT WARNING: Regardless of whether you consider marijuana to be harmful or not, or a "gateway drug" or not, **KEEP ALL FORMS, ESPECIALLY YUMMY EDIBLE FORMS, OUT OF THE REACH OF CHILDREN AND TEENS!** Whether it is raw buds and leaves or brownies, cookies, lollypops, a smoothie or whatever these items MUST be treated as edibles **for adult use only.** You manage to keep truly deadly substance out of kids reach…drain cleaners, insecticides, rat poison, and over-the-counter and prescription drugs…**PLEASE** be equally diligent about **ALL** forms of marijuana.

MARIJUANA – THE WONDER WEED

EVERYTHING YOU NEED TO KNOW
AND WHY IT *MUST* BE LEGALIZED

INDEX

DEDICATIONS

DISCLAIMERS

INTRODUCTION

CHAPTERS

INTRODUCTION

There are a number of reasons for my writing this book. As an advocate for marijuana legalization I hope to provide my readers with a wealth of information on the subject. This book is not written *specifically* to educate. The purpose of information is not education but <u>action</u>. I hope these pages will inspire some to take action and help those of us throughout the nation who are trying our best to lead the battle for marijuana legalization.

It has been said, however, that: "Those convinced by my word against their will shall remain of the same opinion still." It is almost impossible to change the mind of someone who is so inflexible in their beliefs that no amount of facts or proof could possibly change their minds. To those I say: "Thanks for acquiring my book! I hope you find it a fun read."

To those who already support legalization of marijuana.....reportedly 80%+ in favor of medical marijuana, and 50%+ in favor of recreational use, I say: "Thanks for buying my book! I hope it serves to reinforce and validate your opinions."

To all of the others who might not have given the issue a lot of thought, or might not have formed an opinion one way or the other as yet: "Thanks for buying my book! May it serve to give you a sound basis for forming an opinion."

There are six basic goals I considered while writing this book. They are all based on providing enough information for any fair-minded individual to agree:

> 1. To allow industrial hemp cultivation throughout the United States;

2. To re-schedule marijuana to federal Schedule III or better, or remove it from the Schedules entirely the same as alcohol and tobacco;

3. To decriminalize marijuana possession at the federal level;

4. To allow medical marijuana use for virtually any ailment;

5. To allow full recreational use, by treating marijuana exactly the same as alcohol and tobacco;

6. To put ALL marijuana-related decisions in the hands of the several states and territories.

Our Federal Government's attitude towards both marijuana decriminalization and legalization is a shamefull NATIONAL DISGRACE!

What is wrong with most of our politicians? Have they no conscience? Have they no shame at all? Apparently not.

Are they simply *ignorant* of the truth (somewhat forgivable), or are they aware of the truth but totally controlled by the huge pharmaceutical companies ("Big Pharma") with their bottomless treasure chests? Are they so terrified of the controlling federal agencies that they are incapable of rational humanitarian action?

Why have "marijuana-positive-results" in *government* study after study been under-reported or totally dismissed? How can any rational nation classify a natural herb that has been used safely for thousands of years by tens of millions of people in the *same* category as deadly addictive heroin and crack cocaine? Or in a *worse* category than deadly fentanyl? Our government does. **It <u>totally</u> defies logic and reason.**

Why are almost all of our physicians unwilling to prescribe marijuana even in those enlightened states where medical marijuana use is legal? Why is it that naturopathic physicians have no such reservations?

How can our politicians sit on their dead asses idly by as a reported twenty-two heroic American war veterans suffering from Post-Traumatic Stress Disorder, treated with addictive opioids and anti-depressants at the Veterans Administration Hospitals, commit suicide **<u>every day</u>**?

How can anyone of conscience not act to relieve the agony of millions of our citizens who suffer from cancer's ravages, chronic pain, multiple sclerosis, neuropathy, glaucoma, epilepsy, seizures, fibromyalgia, HIV, and a litany of other very serious ailments for which marijuana has been demonstrated, over and over and over, to offer blessed relief?

We are supposed to be "The Land of the Free and the Home of The Brave". We are most assuredly NOT the "Land of the Compassionate". It is truly an unconscionable *National Disgrace*.

Is Senator Bernie Sanders our only remote hope in this battle for legalization?

Why am I particularly passionate about the legalization of marijuana? Why did I start an Arizona non-profit corporation: the National Weed Legalization Fund? TNWLF.org Allow me to explain.

My mother died at age 47 from cirrhosis of the liver caused by alcohol addiction. Alcohol was her way of dealing with an incident where a man committed suicide by jumping off a roof and landing at her feet. She suffered from Post-Traumatic Stress Disorder, the same fate that afflicts so many of our combat veterans.

Alcohol only took three years to kill mom. It makes no sense to me to allow as fully-legal a substance that is known to cause illness and death. Then we ban an amazing healing herb that has thousands of years of documented medicinal value. It makes no sense at all. None.

My closest and dearest friend Joel and I were friends when we were in diapers. We were golf buddies for years, and stayed close throughout our lives. He began smoking at a young age because both of his parents smoked. (Fortunately for me neither of mine did.) He suffered from lung problems all his life. He died of lung cancer many years before his time. Cigarettes kill. Alcohol kills. Marijuana **cures**.

Then there was my wife's mom, the best mother-in-law anyone could wish for. She was a clean living non-smoker who lived on a farm, yet contracted cancer in her late 60s and died at age 71. I watched sadly through her years of chemotherapy and witnessed the constant debilitating nausea caused by the toxic chemical cocktails she was fed. Marijuana is well documented to ease the complications of chemotherapy.

She need not have suffered all of those years. She was simply born too soon. That was the '90s, before anyone in America had the courage to allow medical marijuana *anywhere* to treat nausea caused by chemotherapy.

Next, I am a multiple sclerosis patient. I was diagnosed at Johns Hopkins in 1970 at age 32. I have undergone every MS treatment known to man. I have taken every new "wonder-medicine" as it became available over the years, and absolutely NOTHING helped me in any way I could perceive. Most medicines simply made me feel worse.

I read articles about the many MS afflicted individuals who had remarkable results using marijuana to relieve their symptoms. Once I turned to regular marijuana use almost all my pain and numbness disappeared. My balance greatly improved, and my left-eye pain disappeared. My debilitating nightly spasms vanished. I am able to lead a normal life again! I was even able to win the golfing Gold Medal in the local Senior Olympics a few years ago!

And last, but surely not least, there are our brave military veterans. I am an Army vet and active member of The American Legion Post #66 in Green Valley, Arizona. Fortunately I do not personally suffer from PTSD, but I am in constant contact with many vets who do. **Veterans are the primary reason for my passion to see marijuana universally legalized.**

A large percentage, as many as one in three, of our brave veterans return from battle suffering from PTSD. It was called "Battle Fatigue" in WWI and "Shell Shock" in WWII. How many of these vets will continue a lifetime of suffering **needlessly**, and how many will continue the shameful epidemic of veteran suicides while proposed clinical trials of marijuana are denied or destined to drag on endlessly?

I have spoken to many doctors at Veteran's Administration hospitals. Their hands have been tied. They know that the insane poisonous and addictive cocktails of pain killers and anti-depressants (worth many **billions** of dollars to Big Pharma) they regularly prescribe could be eliminated

5

entirely through marijuana prescriptions. Sadly until very recently, they could not prescribe marijuana to their PTSD patients because they are federal employees and marijuana is federally illegal. They could not even *discuss* marijuana with their patients. **This was an unspeakable tragedy.**

Even worse, in the states where marijuana *is* legal for medical purposes, should a veteran have taken it upon themselves to obtain a "marijuana card" and self-medicate with marijuana outside of the VA, they would be disqualified from being treated for *anything* within the VA system. **This is criminal government insanity.**

Beyond publishing and selling this book, what are my plans to help the legalization cause? First of all, any donations to my Arizona non-profit organization, at my website (TNWLF.org), https://www.thenationalweedlegalizationfund.org, will be donated to the various organizations in key states that are lobbying officials to at least listen to their own citizens and vote accordingly.

Perhaps more important, I hope to send copies of this book to EVERY member of the House of Representatives and Senate, to EVERY Governor, and to key members of certain state legislatures. President Obama will get a special autographed personalized copy!

Copies will also be sent to celebrity marijuana-legalization advocates. Copies will also go to known legalization opponents. I can only pray that enough of these will take the time to read this book and hopefully be favorably influenced by the information herein.

I also plan to send copies to every state and local official that I can identify as legalization opponents. Perhaps one or more might actually soften their position, especially important in states where the citizens are in favor of change.

6

At the start of each Chapter I provide a quote attributed to some famous personality. There are quotes by politicians and musicians, Hollywood actors and talk show hosts, journalists and famous entrepreneurs. These are highly intelligent, articulate individuals. They share many opinions in common: "The war on drugs is lost." "Existing federal marijuana laws are wrong." "Legalization in some form is a no-brainer."

So to summarize, between losing my mom to alcohol, my best friend to lung cancer, watching my mother-in-law suffer needlessly during cancer treatment, my personal experience with multiple sclerosis, and my observations of and discussions with PTSD veterans and their doctors, I have more than ample reason to be passionate about seeing marijuana recognized as the miracle herb that it is. I can only hope and pray that my readers will agree.

CHAPTER 1
THE LONG HISTORY OF MARIJUANA

Walter Cronkite, Ex-Anchor, CBS Evening News:
"Tonight we've seen a war that in its broad outline is not working. It seems to this reporter that the time has come to do what President Hoover did when Prohibition was tearing the nation apart."

Dr. Margaret Mead, author and marijuana advocate:
"Never doubt that a small group of thoughtful, committed citizens can change the world. It is the only thing that ever has."

Virtually every American alive today under 85 or so has been taught nothing but bad things about marijuana. The lies perpetuated for decades by the media, politicians and doctors, driven by the financial interests of the huge pharmaceutical industry ("Big Pharma") and others have taken a solid hold.

It has been said that: "It is far easier to fool the people than to un-fool them." In the case of marijuana legalization nothing could be more true. The people have been fooled for eighty years. Let us pray that *un-fooling* will not take that long.

What to me makes the entire argument against marijuana almost silly is to study and learn from the use of this amazing herbal weed throughout millennia. The favorable evidence is simply overwhelming.

Most Americans are unaware of the very long history of the use of marijuana by people seeking relief from a variety of ills. The oldest confirmed use goes back almost **6,000 years to**

China in 3,750 B.C.E. There was a philosopher-farmer named Shen Nung, who later became a mighty emperor.

He was a benevolent Emperor who cared deeply about the health of his subjects. He taught his people about "ta ma" (marijuana). He collected traditions that had been handed down for centuries so that this medical knowledge could be shared from region to region.

Through years of experimentation he developed plant-based cures that he compiled into an encyclopedia called the *Pen Ts'ao*. This was the world's first reported pharmacopoeia. The female plant was said to possess "yin" energy, the male plant "yang". It was recommended for rheumatism, beriberi, constipation, gout, absentmindedness and many other ailments. Shen Nung is a legend in China to this day.

In 2008 a team of archeologists in China uncovered a tomb from 700 B.C.E. They found over two pounds of marijuana along with the bones of the deceased. The more psychoactive female buds had been selectively collected and buried with the deceased.

Around the year 200 C.E., about eighteen-hundred (1,800!) years ago, Hua To, a Chinese surgeon, developed an anesthesia based on marijuana. He created "ma-yo", a mixture of marijuana resin and rice wine. He used it on his patients during surgery. It is recorded that he performed successful grafts, intestinal resections, and chest incisions while his patients were under the influence of his special herbal anesthetic ma-yo.

Marijuana was used for centuries in Egypt. We know this from a number of papyrus documents that have been discovered. The Ebers, Ramesseum III, Berlin and the

Chester Beatty Medical papyri were written as long ago as 1,700 B.C.E., a mere 3,700 years from today!

Around 300 B.C.E. in India marijuana was used in Ayurvedic medicine for the alleviation of migraine headaches and stomach spasms. It was prescribed as an analgesic, antispasmodic, digestion enhancer, and bladder issues.

At about the same time in Greece, Hippocrates, known as the "Father of Medicine", preached the use of botanicals, including marijuana, to promote good health. The ancient Greeks, to whom we owe much of our culture, documented the use of marijuana for nosebleeds, tapeworm, and earaches, among other ailments.

In Rome, Nero's private physician Dioscorides praised marijuana for its medicinal properties. He named it "cannabis sativa", the name it still bears.

In the second century C.E., Pliny the Elder prescribed marijuana for earaches, cramped joints, gout and burns, among other ailments.

For at least a thousand years, from 800 C.E. throughout the Arab world medieval Arabic physicians' patients relied on marijuana for its diuretic, antiemetic, antiepileptic, anti-inflammatory, pain-killing and antipyretic properties.

After Rome collapsed, Western Civilization receded into the Dark Ages, with suppression of the scientific method. This included herbal medicine, with torture or death a common result for anyone who strayed outside the orthodoxy of the medieval Church. No more marijuana.

In the thirteenth century Ibn Beitar documented the fact that Muslim sailors routinely used marijuana to control seasickness. This allowed them to travel in weather that kept most others in port. It led directly to their conquest of the Mediterranean, and their extended commerce with India and distant Asia.

All during this period in both China and India marijuana use became a staple of medical prescriptions. In the sixteenth century Li Shih-chen wrote the *"Pen T'sao Kang Mu"* a compilation of earlier medical knowledge. He credited marijuana with the power to increase the inner *chi*, stimulate circulation, increase the flow of milk in nursing mothers, and help those stricken with paralysis and many other ailments.

During the European Renaissance the veil of ignorance began to be lifted, hastened by the anatomical work of Leonardo da Vinci. The development of the printing press rapidly spread all manner of knowledge. European explorers, returning from various African trips, reported on the use of marijuana to treat malaria, black-water fever, dysentery, blood poisoning, anthrax and even snake bites!

The Portuguese physician Garcia da Orta travelled to India and studied marijuana medicine intensely. He personally selectively bred several strains. In 1563 he wrote a detailed scientific treatise on marijuana's therapeutic uses.

In 1645 a compendium of knowledge of marijuana's medicinal uses, *"The Compleat Herbal"*, recommended marijuana for hot or dry coughs, jaundice, fluxes, colic, worms, inflammations, gout, knotty joints (i.e., arthritis), hip pains and burns.

In 1794 the *"Edinburgh New Dispensatory"* noted that marijuana had therapeutic benefit for patients stricken with venereal disease and bladder problems.

In 1814 Culpepper published the most complete dissertation on marijuana to that date in his *"Complete Herbal"*. It contained an extensive listing of previous knowledge of the

11

many curative values of marijuana.

When Napoleon invaded Egypt, steeped in Muslim culture, his troops were quickly made aware of the value of inhaling the smoke in the countless hash parlors in the region!

In the early nineteenth century, as Europeans travelled to Africa and Asia on a regular basis, they came more and more in contact with marijuana. Physician Louis Aubert-Roche was one of the first to study the medicinal effects of this natural herbal wonder-plant. His 1840 book described in detail the use of marijuana to treat the plague, typhoid fever, and a long list of other ailments.

Around this same time the British East India Company installed a physician named William B. O'Shaughnessy in Calcutta. He spent years critically studying the effects of cannabis on animals, human patients, and on himself! He *validated* the thousands of years of use in India, and discovered many new medicinal uses.

He successfully relieved the pain of patients with rheumatism. He quieted the convulsions of an infant. He quelled the wrenching muscle spasms of patients with rabies and tetanus, similar to the spasms of epilepsy and multiple sclerosis. O'Shaughnessy may be **the one person most responsible for introducing marijuana to Western medicine.**

In 1854 the **United States** *Dispensatory* actually listed marijuana, noting that: "It has been found to produce sleep, allay spasms, to compose nervous inquietude, and to relieve pain. Complaints to which it has been specifically recommended are neuralgia, gout, tetanus, hydrophobia, cholera, convulsions, spasticity, hysteria, mental depression, insanity and uterine hemorrhage."

YET LESS THAN A HUNDRED YEAR LATER THE UNITED STATES COMPLETELY IGNORED THIS 1854 DOCUMENT, AND BANNED MARIJUANA. THEY CRAFTILY REFERRED TO IT ONLY BY ITS MEXICAN NAME "MARIHUANA". THIS DECEPTION WAS TO SEPARATE IT IN THE MINDS OF THE AMERICAN PUBLIC THAT WAS ACCUSTOMED TO SEEING "CANNABIS" AS AN INGREDIANT IN DOZENS OF POPULAR MEDICINES. "MARIHUANA" WAS AS SUCH COMPLETELY UNKNOWN. THAT UNFORTUNATE BAN IS IN EFFECT TO THIS VERY DAY!

So what exactly happened during that time period? Big Pharma happened. The Devil Anslinger happened. The endless lies happened. (See Chapter 4)

Not long after the United States finally and officially recognized the value of marijuana in 1854, the Smith Brothers (of cough drop fame) obtained a potent extract of the Indica strain of this herbal marvel. It became the basis for countless popular tinctures well into the *early 20th century.*

In England, Queen Victoria's personal physician Sir John Russell Reynolds found marijuana useful in treating menstrual cramps, migraines, neuralgia, epileptic convulsions, and senile insomnia. In his scientific review of marijuana in 1890 he noted: "When pure and administered carefully it **is one of the most potent medicines we possess"**.

With capitalist profits as incentive, by 1896 the major pharmaceutical companies hopped on the bandwagon. In a joint venture Eli Lilly and Parke Davis developed a new Indica strain they called "Cannabis Americana". Soon there were literally dozens of over-the-counter remedies available to the public. These included:

- Eli Lilly's *Dr. Brown's Sedative Tablets; Syrup Tolu Compound; and Syrup Lobelia;*

- Parke Davis's *Casadien; Utroval;* and *Veterinary Colic Mixture;*
- Squib Co.'s *Chlorodyne* and *Collodium;*
- Brown Sequard's *Antineuralgic Pills.*

Unfortunately the death knell for marijuana medicines happened almost overnight. <u>The pharmaceutical companies invented morphine, and the hypodermic needle!</u>

Because cannabinoids are fat soluble and barely water soluble, they could not be injected safely. Morphine, and a host of other quickly invented narcotics were inexpensive to produce, were easily standardized, could be safely injected, and were easily administered by physicians. And they were *hugely* profitable. Big Pharma was born.

In spite of this, when Anslinger and the evil, complicit media and forest-paper baron William Randolph Hearst finally got Congress to outlaw marijuana in 1937 there were still twenty-eight marijuana-based products on the market. These products instantly vanished, as did many of the companies that produced them. (See Chapters 3 and 4)

Soon thereafter the long and slow battle for legalization was about to begin!

In 1958 a beatnik pothead named Neal Cassidy made the serious mistake of offering a joint to an undercover narcotics agent. He spent **two years** incarcerated in San Quinton prison! Poet Allen Ginsberg and other young marijuana advocates were deeply troubled and decided to act.

The first American organization to promote legalization was created in 1964 in San Francisco. "LEMAR", <u>LE</u>galize <u>MAR</u>ijuana, was created by a young hippie named Lowell Eggemeier. He performed an act of civil disobedience by

walking into a police station and lighting up a joint!
Eggemeier's attorney drew up defense briefs based in part on
an earlier favorable study commissioned by New York City
Mayor Fiorello La Guardia.

Allen Ginsberg, the creative poet and avid marijuana user,
picked up on Eggemeier's work, and formed "New York
LAMAR". Ginsberg is quoted as saying: "The universal fear of
marijuana was so great that no one would talk openly about it
on a bus. You couldn't talk about changing the law, much
less about smoking grass, for fear you would be arrested."

In 1966 Ginsberg was inspired to write an article for *Atlantic
Monthly*. It was titled: *"The Great Marijuana Hoax: First
Manifesto To End The Bringdown"*. This began a flood of
public information publications including: *The Marijuana
Papers; The Book Of Grass; Pot: A Handbook of Marijuana;*
and *1In 7: Drugs on Campus*. Ginsberg is perhaps *best*
known for parading around Manhattan displaying pro-
marijuana signs.

In 1969 a new magazine was launched titled: *The Marijuana
Review.* It was started by a guy named Ed Rosenthal and a
partner. (Rosenthal today is a world-renowned author of
many authoritative books on marijuana growing.)

The past forty-seven years have seen many legalization
battles fought and lost. But the relentless pressure by the pro-
legalization crowd has ever so slowly resulted in progress.

The Marijuana Review was distributed by the "Underground
Press Syndicate", run by a guy named Tom Forcade. He and
Ed Rosenthal founded *High Times*, a marijuana-based
magazine that thrives to this day.

In 1971 Hugh Hefner of *Playboy* fame gave a small grant to a young attorney named R. Keith Stroup who formed **NORML**, The National Organization for Reform of Marijuana Laws. Stroup's approach was to attack legalization from a legislative lobbying viewpoint. NORML, and its many state and college chapters nationwide, are a major force lobbying for legalization to this day.

In 1972 in California the first legislative legalization effort anywhere in the United States, known as CMI-72, called for marijuana cultivation for personal use. It was roundly defeated, but marked the first spark in the legalization battle.

There is a story that few know or remember. Back in 1973 a man named Bob Randall found that marijuana helped his glaucoma better than prescription drugs. After being busted for growing his own, he pursued the matter through the courts. Amazingly, in 1976 he became the first American to gain access to medical marijuana since its prohibition!

What is even more incredible is that he was given his marijuana medicine by the federal government for free! The National Institute on Drug Abuse (NIDA) under a program they called "The Compassionate Investigational New Drug Program" provided him, and later a few others, with an abysmally low-grade marijuana. (Apparently that is the same strain available today for any federally sponsored research.)

During the first decade of President Nixon's War On Drugs, a marijuana smuggling operation imported more high-quality marijuana from South and Central America and Asia than has ever been seen before or since! There is a book, *The Underground Empire – Where Crime and Governments Embrace,* written by an investigative journalist named James

Mills. It's 1,100 pages long, and is available today on Amazon used for a dollar! It is a bargain and a great read.

One major topic thread in the book is the details of the exploits of a group known as "Marijuana Incorporated" as they were dubbed in a CBS TV show. They were a group of a dozen or so _non-violent_ young businessmen who ran their marijuana smuggling operation better and more efficiently than most American businesses are run today!

They ONLY smuggled marijuana, NEVER hard drugs. They never carried guns. They carried money! In fact, they had so much money that they were able to bribe every imaginable official on the planet! Heads of state were complicit as well. Money talks. It always has and always will. It does today.

Marijuana, Inc. "owned" individuals in charge of air and water ports of entry. They bought whichever politicians were needed to "turn their backs". It included law enforcement employees wherever and whenever needed.

They were bringing in so much marijuana that they bought a FLEET of HUGE OCEAN FREIGHTERS! As many as four freighter loads A DAY were coming into American ports, each loaded with 100,000 pounds of marijuana.

They generated massive sums of cash, and ploughed it all back into more and more ships and planes, and more and more bribes. They kept little for themselves. Aside from the Americas, Marijuana Inc. brought in product from Thailand, Singapore, Africa, and Holland. Their network of distribution throughout the United States would impress Amazon or FedX! They were unstoppable!

The most fascinating aspect of Mills' story is the years-long attempt to capture the Marijuana, Inc. CEO, the legendary ringleader. He was sort of a modern-day Chapo Guzman.....except he was a calm, quiet, unassuming Jewish guy! Not only was he an absolute business genius and incredible manager, but he was virtually impossible to find and apprehend.

The story is reminiscent of Inspector Javert's obsession in pursuing Jean Valjean, or the FBI's Greg Coleman pursuing Jordan Belfort. Centac was a little-known international police organization. United States Centac Agent Dennis Dayle relentlessly pursued the "marijuana businessman" Donald Steinberg. Dayle is quoted as saying: "If the human mind could think it up, Donald Steinberg could make it work. Centac freely acknowledged Steinberg's genius.

After many years of pursuit Steinberg was eventually located and calmly apprehended. I won't spoil the read because the "how" and "where" is so wonderfully ironic! He was convicted, served his time, and became a thoroughly legitimate and respected businessman thereafter. Because of his complete cooperation with authorities, most of Steinberg's inner circle got probation.

Also in response to President Nixon's "War On Drugs", and the futile Mexico border crackdowns, with the help of Ed Rosenthal's published marijuana growing instructions, marijuana began to be grown illegally nationwide!

In 1985, after years of studying all aspects of marijuana and hemp, Jack Herer, a Rosenthal protégé, published the classic: *The Emperor Wears No Clothes.* This was the first serious public education vehicle in favor of hemp and marijuana legalization.

Over the next few decades, especially in California, various legislative initiatives were proposed. Many new lobby groups formed. In 1996 California's "Compassionate Use Act", Proposition 215, was put on the state ballot. It passed with 54% in favor. **It was the first victory anywhere in the United States for the legalization movement.** It was twenty-four years after that first California initiative failed!

NORML's activities led to the formation of The Marijuana Policy Project (MPP), a D.C. organization focused on changing public policy. It presently has over 25,000 members. Along with NORML it is today a leading legalization advocate. An even larger group has formed, Americans for Safe Access, which now has over 30,000 members!

I am not a particularly avid fan of radio talk show host Glenn Beck, but every so often he comes up with a profound observation. He recently spoke about parallel American societies.

There is the one society that the government wants its citizens to believe is happening. There is the *real* society that is *actually* happening. Reality is often inconvenient to the government. A very inconvenient truth.

When Carrie Nation and the budding Suffragette movement managed to get President Wilson and his Progressive allies to agree to alcohol prohibition in the "nation's best interest", we witnessed fourteen years of Beck's parallel societies.

We had the one society the government pretended existed. They did their best to convince the public that it did actually exist. But we also had **reality**! Reality was speakeasies, home brewing, black-market liquor, and as much alcohol consumption as ever, if not more. In addition we introduced rampant organized crime on a scale never before seen.

Beck pointed out something I had never heard before. Apparently the government intentionally poisoned liquor supplies and killed 50,000 citizens during prohibition! The rationale was: "Alcohol is going to kill them anyway so what's the difference?" They wanted to be certain prohibition lasted. Of course it didn't. Could this be true? Beck says it is. Conspiracy theorists rejoice!

Having learned nothing from alcohol prohibition, or not giving a damn, Anslinger and Hearst managed to create another eighty years of parallel societies. We have the marijuana-free utopia with the federal government trying its best to ignore the medical value of marijuana and its use everywhere, and we have reality. Reality is that marijuana is more available than ever, and the War On Drugs is a total failure.

Through prohibition, and suppression of the truth about marijuana, the government has succeeded in keeping the illusion alive, while **reality** is quite the opposite! It has also succeeded in killing legions of its citizens once again.

Beck skipped over the marijuana issue entirely and went on to point out that we have two parallel entertainment societies. One is the politically correct, watered-down-language, no full-frontal-nudity plain-vanilla network TV show society.

The other is the **reality** society in which we all curse and openly hate whomever we chose and turn to the TV programming (Game of Thrones comes to mind) where the real society, with all of its gritty faults, filthy language and every-day nudity is fully exposed.

The marijuana charade cannot, *must not*, go on forever!
The road to legalization *started* thousands of years ago in
China! With the help of all of the many pro-legalization lobby
groups, and the support of educated Americans, let's hope the
road *ends* In America, sooner than later.

.

CHAPTER 2
AMERICA'S MARIJUANA CULTURE

Tony Bennett, Singer, Grammy Winner:
"I'd like to have every gentleman and lady in this room commit themselves to get our government to legalize drugs -- so they'll have to get it through a doctor, not just some gangsters that just sell it under the table."

The entire matter of The War On Drugs and the entire matter of legalization and rescheduling of marijuana is a sick joke. Marijuana has been an integral part of American culture for over a hundred years. Marijuana has infused itself into our movies, and even more so into our music. That is fact.

Beyond that, a subject that is almost NEVER discussed in the media is the almost *universal* use of marijuana in American colleges. I'm not just talking about students. You can include professors, deans, administrators, maintenance workers and even coaches among the ranks of regular users.

One of my kids attended college. Most of my friend's kids attended college. The stories of dorm use of marijuana all match.....marijuana smokers are in the majority! All also mentioned many instances of their professors joining in! *High Times Magazine* each year does a careful study of American Colleges. They list the year's top ten of these pillars of higher education in terms of per-student marijuana use.

There is a national lobby organization, *Students for Sensible Drug Policy (SSDP)* that has active chapters on almost all campuses. Many colleges also have chapters of the huge national organization NORML (The National Organization for Reform of Marijuana Laws) on their campuses.

22

In fact, it is very likely that much of the progress that has been made in recent years in the legalization effort has been the result of the lobbying of these student groups nationwide. Colleges that are reported to have particularly active lobby groups include:

- The University of Michigan, Ann Arbor
- Brown University, Providence, Rhode Island
- University of Connecticut, Storrs
- The University of Maryland, College Park
- Roosevelt University, Chicago
- American University, Washington, DC
- Franklin Pierce University, Ridge, New Hampshire
- University of Central Florida, Orlando
- Missouri Southern State University, Joplin
- The University of Memphis, Tennessee

This list, however, is barely the tip of the marijuana campus iceberg! It would be difficult, if not impossible to find any college where an active pro-legalization group of some size does not flourish, and marijuana use is uncommon.

Let us not forget Great Britain's oldest and most prestigious college, Oxford. This is where President Bill Clinton in 1968, a brilliant Rhodes Scholar, famously "didn't inhale"! Marijuana use in college is certainly not prevalent *only* in the good old US of A.

Let's take a look at Hollywood. Since 1968 there have been well over a dozen popular marijuana-themed flicks including:

- I Love You, Alice B. Toklas (1968) (NOTE: Alice B. Toklas was famous for publishing a cannabis-infused brownie recipe in the 1920s!)
- Easy Rider (1969)

- Fritz The Cat (1972)
- Up In Smoke (1978)
- Apocalypse Now (1979)
- Dazed and Confused (1993)
- Friday (1995)
- Half Baked (1998)
- The Big Lebowski (1998)
- How High (2001)
- Harold & Kumar Go To White Castle (2004)
- Grandma's Boy (2006)
- Super high Me (2007)
- Pineapple Express (2008)
- Humboldt County (2008)
- We're The Millers (2013)
- This Is The End (2013)

Beyond Hollywood films, there have been many very popular bands and vocalists whose music often related in some way to drugs or marijuana.

Marijuana music has evolved over the years from the jazz of the first half of the 20th century, through rock and roll during the "Flower Power" '60s, then to heavy metal, progressive rock, Jamaican reggae in the 70s to the hip-hop, jam bands and rap music of the present day.

The first popular marijuana song was recorded by a young Louis Armstrong in 1929, "*Muggles*", which was marijuana slang of the day. Other jazz greats composed hits such as Cab Calloway's "*Reefer Man*" and Benny Goodman's "*Texas Tea Party*". After prohibition in 1937, songs such as C. P. Johnson's "*The G Man Got the T Man*" became popular.

But it wasn't until the '60s when Bob Dylan led the marijuana counter-culture charge with the ever popular "*Mr. Tambourine Man*" and "*Rainy Day Woman*", the latter with its memorable chorus: "Everybody must get stoned." In that same era David Peel recorded "*I Like Marijuana*" in 1968.

It was during this era that poet Alan Ginsberg marched around New York City with his pro-marijuana signs!

Other well-known popular music included:

- Pink Floyd ("*The Wall*"; "*Dark Side Of The Moon*")
- The Beatles ("*Strawberry Fields Forever*", "*Lucy In The Sky With Diamonds*")
- The Grateful Dead ("*Uncle John's Band*"; "*Sugar Magnolia*")
- Jefferson Airplane ("*Mexico*")
- Bob Marley and The Wailers ("*Kaya*")
- Peter Tosh ("*Legalize It*")
- Cypress Hill ("*I Wanna Get High*"; "*Hits From The Bong*")
- Snoop Dog ("*Gin and Juice*")
- The Doors ("*Riders On The Storm*"; "*The End*"; "*Light My Fire*")
- Aerosmith ("*Reefer Head Woman*")
- Rush ("*A Passage To Bangkok*")
- Black Sabbath ("*Sweet Leaf*"; "*It's So Nice To Be Stoned*")
- Jim Safford ("*Wildwood Weed*")
- John Denver ("*Rocky Mountain High*")
- Peter, Paul & Mary ("*Puff The Magic Dragon*")
- The Association ("*Along Comes Mary*")

Recently, hip-hop and rap artists have created hundreds of marijuana songs. Artists such as Snoop Dog, Dr. Dre, Wiz

Khalifa, Kool Keith and Del the Funky Homosapien have led the charge. The list goes on and on!

In 1971 a group of students from San Rafael High School in California created a code term: "4:20", "420" or "4/20". It was the time of day for their "secret" meetings on school grounds. Since then, "four twenty" has referred to marijuana smoking in general. April 20th is considered National Marijuana Day!

Every year there are marijuana festivals throughout the United States. Starting back in April 1972 the "Hash Bash" annual event was held in Ann Arbor, Michigan.

The "Seattle Hempfest" (formerly The Washington Hemp Expo) began in 1991, and attracts hundreds of thousands of marijuana devotees every year.

Portland, Oregon has an annual "Hempstalk" festival the second weekend in September at Kelly Point Park where the Willamette and Columbia Rivers come together.

And of course there are periodic music festivals where marijuana smoking is generally tolerated. The most famous festival, attended by an estimated 400,000, happened in Woodstock, New York on August 17, 1969. One could conclude that this was the beginning of the national legalization movement.

Here is **_a little known fact_** that qualifies as "American Culture". During World War II, the American military used heavy doses of marijuana as an *interrogation vehicle* on enemy prisoners! Apparently it was very effective. I wonder how its effectiveness compares to water-boarding?

In spite of all of the horrible media attention, the lobbying of Big Pharma, and clueless or bought-off politicians and doctors, marijuana has been a large part of mainstream American culture for **_decades_**.

Finally, after so many years, the legalization movement is making real progress.

It has not been an easy road.

CHAPTER 3
THE FEDERAL WAR ON DRUGS

Pat Robertson, Founder of the Christian Broadcasting Network:
"I really believe we should treat marijuana the way we treat beverage alcohol. I've never used marijuana and I don't intend to, but it's just one of those things that I think: this war on drugs just hasn't succeeded."

Shepard Smith, Host of Fox News Channel's "Fox Report":
"If there's a war on drugs, it's lost. Bring everyone home, because the war on drugs is over... End the war. This is stupid. This is a stupid war, isn't it? We've lost this war. This war is lost."

Brad Pitt, Hollywood Actor and Producer:
"We have spent a trillion dollars. It's lasted for over 40 years. A lot of people have lost their lives for it. It's an incredible failure. The drug war is actually being used to hold a portion of our society down. It's criminal in itself. The only way to end the war on drugs is to take the profit out of it. We have to look at the "what-if-everything-was-legal" and people were allowed to make their own choices... If you decriminalize, then they could control the quality. And I propose you would have fewer deaths."

Sting, The late Grammy, Emmy and Golden Globe Award-Winning Musician:
"The War on Drugs has failed -- but it's worse than that. It is actively harming our society. Violent crime is thriving in the shadows to which the drug trade has been consigned. People who genuinely need help can't get it.

We are spending billions, filling up our prisons with non-violent offenders and sacrificing our liberties. Literally hundreds of billions of dollars -- dollars denied to urgent problems ranging from poverty to pollution, have been spent and wasted. People who *do* need help with drugs have been treated as criminals instead."

THE ABOVE ARE NOT THE WORDS OF STUPID PEOPLE! READ THEM, AND PLEASE BELIEVE THAT WHAT THEY SAY IS RIGHT ON TARGET!

In 1986 James Mills copyrighted, and Doubleday published, the aforementioned 1100+ page book: *"The Underground Empire – Where Crime and Governments Embrace".* It is readily available in used condition today on Amazon. It is highly suggested reading because of its current relevance to the endless discussions of the legalization of marijuana.

Marijuana, Inc. ended its activities with the conviction and incarceration of its leader. This was after a decade of expending vast government resources pursuing a small number of individuals central to the operation. Was anything actually accomplished? Was the war on drugs won? Did anything material actually change? Of course not.

In fact, the void caused by the shutdown of Marijuana Incorporated was quickly filled by the infamous Black Tuna Gang operation in the 1980s.

What appears to always be underestimated by our government is the almost unlimited power of really BIG-money to corrupt virtually anyone on any level. Illegal marijuana is BIG money. Legal prescription drugs are BIGGER money. Big Pharma earns billions selling *legal,* government approved, deadly addictive drugs. Do *they* have the money to lobby and corrupt? Of course they do.

The Underground Empire clearly documents that no level of authority is immune to bribes. This includes everyone from politicians and judges, law enforcers, sea, land and air carriers, to dock and airport authorities. It is well documented that entire *countries* are "owned" by drug cartels.

Mill's book, written over thirty years ago, ended with a prophetic paragraph. After concluding his chronicle with the government at long last closing down "Marijuana Inc.", Mills ended with his brilliant observation of the moment:

"Cocaine and marijuana were on the move, and across the continent and a couple of ocean poppies thrived unmolested. Hundreds of billions of dollars were coursing into vast unseen oceans of wealth --- a few drops trickling away to buy weapons, hire terrorists, corrupt governments, subvert nations. *And in Washington someone was no doubt planning another media campaign to tell us of the latest offensive in the war on drugs.* **The Underground Empire was alive and flourishing.**" (Emphases mine.)

Who came up with the term: "The War On Drugs"? Why it was none other than President Nixon, "Tricky Dick", who coined it. After the courts earlier essentially weakened Anslinger's personal war against marijuana, Nixon set up "The Shafer Commission" which to his dismay recommended decriminalization!

The report concluded: **"Neither the marihuana user nor the drug itself can be said to constitute a danger to public safety."** Nixon is reported to have been beyond furious! In response he declared a federal "**War On Drugs**" that continues to this very day.

30

Nixon apparently exploded into quite a rant! It seems he hated Jews as much as he hated marijuana. H. R. Haldeman, Nixon's Chief of Staff, revealed a recording he had made. On it, Nixon is heard saying: "I want a Goddamn strong statement on marijuana that just tears the ass out of them. Every one of those bastards who are for legalizing marijuana is Jewish."

"What the Christ is wrong with the Jews, Bob? What is the matter with them? I suppose it's because most of them are psychiatrists, you know, there's so many, all the great psychiatrists are Jewish. We are going to hit the marijuana thing, and I want to hit it right square in the puss." Nice rant, Tricky Dick. Anslinger blamed "The Negroes". Nixon blamed "The Jews". Both of them were utter fools.

President Jimmy Carter was a bit more enlightened. Speaking about marijuana, he told Congress: "Penalties against possession of a drug should not be more damaging to an individual than the use of the drug itself; and where they are, they should be changed". Of course Congress didn't listen!

The fact is, only through real *financial disincentive* can any progress on the drug war ever be made. And there is one very simple potential financial disincentive.....**LEGALIZE MARIJUANA!**

Although legalizing marijuana in many states has not yet been shown for sure to create such a disincentive, it definitely could in the future. The "Colorado Experiment" is proving that *over-regulation* of legal marijuana creates a legal-marijuana pricing-model that ends up giving the illegal distributors and cartels an opening for a major pricing advantage.

Those many I have interviewed, each with extensive experience in growing marijuana, know with *certainty* that in the future, with intelligent regulation, the black market in marijuana can be smoked (pun intended!). ***If only Washington would listen to the industry professionals.***

Hundreds of millions, perhaps billions, of taxpayer dollars have been spent on anti-marijuana propaganda advertisements, both TV and radio. These were not only tragically misleading, some were downright funny!

We all remember that Nancy Reagan coined the phrase: "Just Say No". Most said "Yes"! She had a profound influence over her husband. I consider Ronald Reagan to have been one of our most effective presidents ever overall. Sadly he wasn't perfect. Far from it.

President Reagan made the most *ludicrous* statement about marijuana in human history: "I now have absolute proof that smoking even one marijuana cigarette is equal in brain damage to being on Bikini Island during an H-bomb blast." Seriously Ronny? Well at least they wouldn't be picking you up with a blotter!

What is our generally undereducated public (Rush Limbaugh refers to them as the "low information crowd") to believe when the leader of the free world makes a statement like that? Truly reprehensible. Shame on Reagan.

Among the earliest anti-marijuana ads was one featuring Sonny Bono. After scenes of various teens smoking pot and getting high, a dude in a leather jacket drives an old jalopy down a hill, jumps out while the car is moving, and of course the car crashes…fade to black. Sonny then slowly recites how marijuana will destroy your teenage years and take all of the meaning from your life! Really?

In the late '80s a series of ads aired using the theme: "I learned it by watching you." The punch line was: " Parents who use drugs have children who use drugs." Of course the same can be said about parents who use tobacco and alcohol, and eat pizza.

In the wake of the 9-11 terrorist attack in New York City, The Office of National Drug Control Policy (ONDCP) debuted a series of TV ads that linked drug use with supporting terrorists! A teen age boy facing the camera says: "I killed mothers. I killed fathers. I killed grandmas. I killed grandpas. I killed sons. I killed daughters." He continues with: "Drug money supports terror. If you buy drugs you will too." You can't make this stuff up.

Later in 2002 the same ONDCP group launched its "They'll Understand" campaign. In one ad a toddler drops a toy into a swimming pool and drowns trying to retrieve it. Sweet. The narrator says: "Just tell her parents you weren't watching her because you were getting stoned. They'll understand." Gag!

In 2006 the same group of geniuses unveiled a series of "dog shaming" cartoons. The recurring theme is the dog's disappointment with its owner for smoking marijuana. Nothing like being shamed by Fido! In another ad the guy tries to get the dog to try a joint. The dog refuses in disgust. Touching.

Not to be upstaged by a pooch, in yet another ad from the series the guy's girlfriend replaces the pup. He lights up a joint, and she says: "Not again!" And then, as if by magic, a marijuana-free alien spaceship swoops down and sweeps the girl off her feet! You REALLY cannot make this stuff up.

The government itself actually did a study of the ONDCP's ads and concluded that the ads clearly made many groups of kids **_actually try marijuana for the first time_**! This was during the Bush administration. The study was kept under wraps for years until it was finally leaked to the public.

And let us not forget the more recent: "This is your brain on drugs!" ads featuring a truly disgusting runny and gross looking sunny side up egg after being dropped on a hot griddle and instantly fried. I haven't eaten an egg since!

Overall the government has wasted untold BILLIONS of taxpayer dollars in a futile attempt to win the War On Drugs. Obviously we need to try something new and different.

Any of the deadly street drugs kids take today (see Chapter23) can be bought by any pre-teen or teen who makes even a modest effort to find it. I don't care if it is in an affluent city, a ghetto, or a farm community, these drugs can be bought *everywhere*. <u>Some can even be bought over the counter or on the internet!</u>

The deluge of toxic street drugs, hyperventilating media coverage, and a recent huge increase in hospitalizations and deaths have shattered forever *any* illusion that Nixon's War has been won on any level.

Recently, New York, Mississippi and Alabama have all issued state health alerts following a dramatic rise in street drug overdoses. Arizona, Florida, New Jersey and Texas report a similar surge.

The basic problem is that corrupt , sophisticated PhD chemists in China, India and Pakistan and elsewhere can tweak the chemical constituents of "designer drugs" faster than law enforcement can even classify them as illegal. This makes the War On Drugs harder to win than the war on ISIS.

One of the invariable unintended consequences of the War On Drugs is referred to as "substance displacement". The United Nations Office on Drugs and Crime point out that when you control one drug successfully it simply causes users and suppliers to move on to a different drug with similar or worse effects by having no controls whatsoever.

They also note that after any successes in the enforcement of the *supply* side of a street drug the *demand* remains the same and the drug entrepreneurs move in to supply that demand with something new and often even *more* deadly.

Remember Obama's recent: "Let's try something new" remark, referring to Cuban relations? Here's a great new suggestion: Decriminalize marijuana. Un-classify marijuana, or reclassify it to Schedule III. Let's try something new! Duh.

To date the "War On Drugs" has clearly been lost. The government cannot deny this, despite the untold billions of dollars wasted yearly. Can this war ever be won? Perhaps, perhaps not.

If the government would just have the basic common sense to decriminalize and legalize marijuana and focus all of those vast wasted resources on stopping the truly dangerous designer street drugs and conventional cocaine and heroin it could *only* be a major step in the right direction.

As mentioned above, President Obama earlier in 2016 paid an historic visit to Cuba. Although many criticized the visit, he said something quite profound as the reason for his visit: "We've tried the same Cuban policy for fifty years and it hasn't worked. *It's time to try something new.*" **BINGO! Let's apply that logic to the totally failed War On Drugs.**

Suggestion: Make marijuana universally available just as alcohol and tobacco is universally available. Let the states and territories decide on everything of this nature, consistent with our great Constitution.

Give marijuana a few years to stabilize in the marketplace. Create hundreds of thousands of new jobs. Collect massive tax revenues. Save billions on law enforcement and prisons.

After this, evaluate whether marijuana actually replaces the vastly more dangerous addictive substances, greatly reduces deaths, and in general makes for a happier and more laid-back American society.

You might just be surprised at the sum of all of the results!

CHAPTER 4
REQUIEM: THE DEVIL ANSLINGER

Ann Druyan, Author, Producer, widow of Carl Sagan:
"I really believe that the marijuana laws are a terrible injustice. They make no sense scientifically, ethically, legally or any way. They cost a fortune to enforce and we incarcerate hundreds of thousands of people who have done nothing else but possess or distribute marijuana."

Do you know a lot about Harry Jacob Anslinger? Probably not, unless you are ninety-plus years old and lived during alcohol prohibition.

The 18th Amendment to the United States Constitution, prohibiting the sale and consumption of alcoholic beverages was passed in January 1920. It was finally repealed by the 21st Amendment in December 1933. **Fourteen years of abysmal failure** was enough. Eliot Ness and his "Untouchables" were a waste of taxpayer money. (Sort of reminds one of Nixon's War On Drugs!)

Harry J. Anslinger was the assistant Commissioner of the United States Bureau of Prohibition. As prohibition was winding down he was appointed head of the shiny new Treasury Department's "Federal Bureau of Narcotics" (FBN) in 1930.

After prohibition ended, Anslinger still had a good job as FBN Head. The problem was, he and his new Bureau had virtually nothing to do! Don't worry, be happy....**he simply made something up to keep his job relevant!** He desperately needed a Boogie Man, and there was one just waiting in the wings. It was cannabis. He called it "MARIHUANA".

Over the years, and during prohibition, Anslinger had been

quoted as saying that "cannabis" (it was only known as such at that time) was totally harmless. Of course he knew that it was used in dozens of effective medicines and had been popular since the late 1890s. He is even quoted as saying that it was a "fallacy" that it caused violence in its users.

Whoops! Quickie change of heart. Sudden 180 in 1930! Job security and all that rot. He unexplainably became marijuana's Public Enemy #1! His evil legacy continues to this day, not just in America but worldwide.

Anslinger spoke publically about the many evils of marijuana. He spoke of wild eroticism, boggled thought processes, maddening nightmares, and eventual total insanity. He called it the "Demon Weed", and scared the Holy crap out of the American public. He essentially blamed blacks, Mexicans, other minorities and jazz musicians for the "problem".

He had read a story about a young boy who hacked his entire family to death. Anslinger warned every parent in the country that a similar fate would befall them if their kid ever smoked marihuana. Who wants to be chopped up in their sleep by a marihuana-crazed kid? Not many. He made certain that every media outlet of the day featured this story. And they did.

Some years later someone tracked down the medical records of the child axe-murderer. The horrific act actually did take place. But it was discovered that there existed absolutely NO EVIDENCE WHATSOEVER that could be found showing that the kid was *ever* exposed to *any* marijuana! He had a family history of mental illness and violence, and his family had been told for years that he should be institutionalized. WOW!

Check out Chapter 8 and the sad sensational story about "Little Jimmy" and a rescinded Pulitzer Prize. It is criminal that we can all be misled by totally fabricated media propaganda. It is why so many in this country both loath and fear our media *and* our politicians and their selfish motives. Years of lies have taken their toll. Isn't this why Donald Trump is so popular?

A job- desperate Anslinger canvassed doctor after doctor and finally found ONE, just one, out of the dozens he contacted, that said marijuana *might* be dangerous. **Success!** (The rest of the doctors said *marijuana was absolutely harmless!*) So, armed with his new doctor/scientist/expert ally and the axe-wielding kid as proof positive of the evils of marihuana he and a media accomplice terrorized the country for years.

To make matters worse, The Bureau of Narcotics had yet another ally. He was the money-hungry co-conspirator , the wealthy and powerful media mogul William Randolph Hearst. He had wisely invested heavily in the timber industry to support his massive newspaper empire's insatiable appetite for wood pulp and paper. He became Anslinger's top accomplice.

To Hearst, the very idea of marihuana/hemp-fiber-based competition was unthinkable. So he agreed to publish in his vast newspaper chain **every line of filth about marihuana that Anslinger could make up.** It was the perfect marriage of a greedy industrialist and a man on a job-saving mission.

Here is a small sample of Anslinger's totally fabricated lies that Hearst eagerly printed:

"Marihuana is an addictive drug which produces in its users insanity, criminality and death".

"You smoke just one joint and you are likely to kill your brother". (I guess it was OK if you were an only child or if you only had a sister.)

"Marihuana is the most violence-causing drug in the history of mankind."

"The primary reason to outlaw marihuana is its effect on the degenerative races". Anslinger despised *anyone* who wasn't white. They were *all* degenerates!

"There are 100,000 total marihuana smokers in the U. S., and most are Negroes, Hispanics, Filipinos and entertainers. Their Satanic music, jazz, and swing, result from marihuana use."

"This marihuana causes white women to seek sexual relations with Negroes, entertainers and any others". I assume the "others" were the Filipinos and Hispanics!

"Reefers make "darkies" think they are as good as white men". He must have been a Stephen Foster fan!

"Colored students at the University of Minnesota, partying with white female students, smoking marihuana and getting their sympathy with stories of racial persecution.....Result: pregnancy." Those must have been *damn* good stories!

"Two Negroes took a girl of fourteen years old and kept her for two days under the influence of marihuana. Upon recovery she was found to be suffering from syphilis."

In addition to the above absurd and <u>totally fabricated</u> and published quotes, Hearst's newspapers blasted out front page headlines such as:

"MARIHUANA MAKES FIENDS OF BOYS IN THIRTY DAYS!"

"MARIHUANA GOADS USERS TO BLOODLUST!"

"MARIHUANA INFLUENCED NEGROES TO LOOK AT WHITE PEOPLE IN THE EYE, STEP ON WHITE MEN'S SHADOWS, AND LOOK AT A WHITE WOMAN TWICE!" That shadow stuff is *really* scary!

"MARIHUANA IS RESPONSIBLE FOR THE RAPING OF WHITE WOMEN BY CRAZED NEGROES!"

"THREE FORTHS OF THE CRIMES OF VIOLENCE IN THIS COUNTRY TODAY ARE COMMITTED BY MARIHUANA SLAVES. THAT IS A MATTER OF COLD RECORD."

Just reading this crap, written by a high federal public official, certainly gives one a better understanding of just how deep-rooted racial prejudices must have been planted in Whites' minds before national desegregation.

People must have read these headlines and, as people tend to do today, believe as fact the many media lies and distortions. They simply accept this garbage as FACT. *Very few ever took the time to seek the truth.* Of course, without the internet and Google, social media, and Wikipedia, truth-seeking-research was virtually impossible anyway.

Reading this garbage today, in our much more enlightened and informed society, some of it is almost amusing. But just as the lies about marijuana stuck in the collective consciousness of decades of Americans, so must have the denigration of minorities by Anslinger and Hearst contributed to the deep-rooted racial hatreds of those days.

This stuff is so outrageous that it seems impossible for a nation to be convinced for eighty-plus years to ban a harmless herbal medicine. Sadly, it was not at all impossible.

This is the stuff my parents were subjected to (I was born in 1938) and probably actually believed. Not even today's most ardent anti-marijuana advocates or avowed racists would consider any of this nonsense to have the slightest hint of validity. At least I hope not.

Corporate greed seemingly has no bounds. DuPont

Chemical happily joined the Anslinger/Hearst conspiracy. With his own propaganda papers widely accepted, and the weight of a mega-corporation behind his efforts, in 1937 Anslinger presented his "Marijuana Tax Act" to Congress.

It was passed with almost no debate. It effectively prohibited marijuana use, sale and growth in the United States to this very day. Anslinger's years-long brainwashing campaign had succeeded. It also immediately put over thirty cannabis-medicine manufacturers out of business, and dashed the hopes of anyone growing industrial hemp.

Anslinger and Hearst did one thing that was incredibly clever. They NEVER referred to "cannabis" or "hemp". "Cannabis" had been firmly fixed in Americans' minds as the primary ingredient in dozens of popular and effective medicines for decades.

The general public totally failed to grasp that the "evil Mexican marihuana" referred to in the new law and in all of Anslinger's ravings and Hearst's newspapers was THE VERY SAME CANNABIS PLANT that had been effectively used as medicine, in religious ceremonies, and for pleasure, for many thousands of years!

Hemp had been used for centuries for a variety of useful items (See Chapter 12). Virtually no one made the connection between the familiar "cannabis" or "hemp" with the new hyper-evil "Mexican Marihuana" threat.

Anslinger and Hearst purposely kept the Mexican spelling (with an h in the middle instead of a j) to connect it directly with the "filthy, despicable, to-be-hated Mexicans" who were bringing this evil menace across the border. Their lies were creative, and endless:

"By the tons it is coming into this country ---- the deadly

dreadful poison that racks and tears not only the body but the very heart and soul of every human being who once becomes a slave to it in any of its cruel and devastating forms."

"Marijuana is a short cut to the insane asylum. Smoke marihuana cigarettes for a month and what was once your brain will be nothing but a storehouse of horrid specters. Marihuana makes a murderer who kills for the love of killing out of the mildest mannered man who ever laughed at the idea that any habit could ever get him."

I'll say one thing for Anslinger and Hearst. They sure could write great imaginary propaganda!

My maternal grandmother was born in 1886, and seemed to me to live forever! She credited her longevity to a pack of cigarettes and a half-bottle of Scotch a day. Whatever. Her maiden name was "Tilden", a close relative of Samuel J. Tilden who ran for the presidency, won the popular vote, and lost a contested Democrat Convention! Sound familiar?

Whenever I was ill as a child grandma used to tell me about the wonderful cannabis medicines that her family had relied heavily on since the turn of the century. She never quite understood why "they simply stopped making them" after 1937! Thank you again, Harry Anslinger.

Arguably the greatest mayor in the history of New York City, the legendary Fiorello La Guardia, decided to commission a study of the effects of smoking marihuana.

His "La Guardia Committee", assembled in 1939, was America's first in-depth study of "marihuana". Their conclusions, after five years of intense study, systematically contradicted **all** of the claims made by Anslinger and the U. S. Treasury Department. No, marihuana did not result in insanity. No, it was not addictive. It was a proven medicine.

The Committee determined that: "The practice of smoking marihuana does not lead to physical addiction in the medical sense of the word." Released in 1944, the report infuriated Anslinger who of course condemned it as "unscientific" and smeared it on every possible occasion in Hearst's press..

Was Anslinger content with his success at banning marijuana in the United States? Hell no! After achieving his goals in America he drafted the United Nations "Single Convention On Narcotic Drugs". In 1954 he saw to it that almost all member nations signed it.

The end result of Anslinger's hatred of all things marijuana is that countless millions worldwide over the past six decades have suffered excessive pain and nausea and many have died needlessly. Marijuana mitigates pain. It reduces epileptic seizures. It can help avoid suicides. Marijuana cures. It has been proven to be a very safe and effective medicine.

As mentioned earlier, President Nixon had a serious bug up his ass about marijuana. Perhaps it had to do with his Quaker upbringing. Do Quakers hate both marijuana *and* Jews? I haven't a clue.

Almost every Presidential term from then on just saw more of the same. One exception was an enlightened Jimmy Carter who strongly endorsed decriminalization. In a speech to Congress he said: "Penalties against possession of a drug should not be more damaging to an individual than the use of the drug itself, and where they are, they should be changed." No one listened or cared.

President William Jefferson Clinton once famously said that he tried marijuana once as a student at Oxford University but did not inhale. At least President Obama, to his credit, when asked if he inhaled replied: "Of course I did. That was the whole idea!"

In 2006 a young man named Mason Tvert got a brilliant idea. Few have ever heard of him. At the time the governor of Colorado was John Hickenlooper. It just so happened that Hickenlooper had made his fortune selling massive amounts of alcohol in pubs across the state. Tvert challenged his governor to a duel! Not exactly an Aaron Burr type duel, but it had as much if not greater effect.

Tvert challenged Hickenlooper to sit down at a table and take a drink of whiskey. Then he would in turn take a marijuana hit. On, and on, and on, until one of them dropped dead! The duel never took place.

Tvert went on to be the #1 advocate for legalization of marijuana in Colorado. Eventually his fellow citizens voted 54.96% to 45.04% to allow full use of marijuana for ANY PURPOSE! This was a bold experiment, and it is now being followed daily by most states in the union to see what problems might occur.

Tvert was well aware that alcohol kills 40,000 Americans every year. Marijuana has **NEVER**, throughout human history, **ever killed anyone!** (Singer Willie Nelson does tell a story about a friend who was killed when a heavy bale of marijuana fell on his head! I don't think that counts.)

As my candidate for "Most Misguided Award Of The Century" I offer the following: In 1958 the National Civil Service League voted Harry J. Anslinger: "One of the ten outstanding government career men." It's all in the viewpoint.

The entire Anslinger episode is a prime example of how the "Big Lie" and repeated unsubstantiated fabricated propaganda (think Adolph Hitler) can change the world for all humanity for many decades.

WE SIMPLY MUST PERMANENTLY REVERSE THIS IDIOCY!

In my opinion Harry Jacob Anslinger may have been the most evil man that ever lived. He was an avowed racist, and helped perpetuate racist feelings for decades. By denying millions worldwide legal access to *Marijuana – The Wonder Weed* he was responsible for more suffering and deaths over the past 79 years than Joseph Stalin and Adolph Hitler combined!

Hearst died on August 14, 1951 at the age of 88.   Anslinger died on January 14, 1975 at 83. One can only hope they both reside in a special place in Hell.

CHAPTER 5
THE BATTLES WE MUST FACE

Jon Stewart, TV Personality, Comedian & Actor:
"I don't think marijuana should be illegal."

There are three fundamental battles that must be recognized in our discussions of the legalization of cannabis:

1. Documenting the safety and efficacy of marijuana itself, especially in comparison to alcohol and tobacco;

2. Educating the general public of the truth as opposed to the lies that are supported by the strong and wealthy special interest lobby groups against legalization;

3. **Deciding how and by whom marijuana should be regulated.**

Each of these battles is one for potentially endless discussion, endless study, and endless disagreement. Yet, with persistence, steady progress has been and continues to be made. Full legalization seems achievable within a few years.

The only *short-term* resolution of "1." is to accept as fact thousands of years of evidence from literally millions of users. Then legalize marijuana on the basis of reason and compassion. Later do whatever "research" makes various interest groups feel warm and fuzzy! As pointed out later in Chapter 10, there are simply too many marijuana variants to make scientific study of every strain and every disease absolutely impossible.

We *CAN* win the battle in "2.". Samuel Clemens (Mark Twain) famously said: "It is extremely easy to fool the people but it is damn near impossible to un-fool them". The public has been fooled for decades regarding the many values of marijuana. This is where groups such as my non-profit National Weed Legalization Fund (NWLF.org) and many larger lobby groups such as NORML are ***absolutely essential.***

It is only through the collective voice (read "collective *funds*") of members of the general public that Big Pharma and other anti-marijuana lobby groups can be defeated. And defeat them we must. But "3."? Well folks, here is where we face the most difficult challenge.

Whether it is on the state level, or the federal level, our system of government, for all its greatness, has one near-fatal flaw. There are simply too many conflicting and overlapping interests that must somehow get into agreement regarding anything affecting the public. They seldom actually do. Endless delay is the resulting order of the day.

Each group will have individuals on either side of "1." and "2." Any one group can cause endless delay or completely stop almost anything from being accomplished. And yet somehow they will all have to play nicely together in the marijuana sandbox if full legalization is to *ever* become a reality. Is this a realistic hope?

For starters, we have our "checks and balances" bicameral system on both the federal and state levels, that is, a House of Representatives and a Senate. Either one at either level can kill any bill by simply not even bringing it up for a vote. But let's assume we can actually get past *that* hurdle. Now the *real* turf battles begin.

On the federal level we have the Drug Enforcement Agency, the Department of Health, The Commodity Trading

48

Commission, the Securities and Exchange Commission, and the Internal Revenue Service , plus GOD knows how many others, all of whom will want some say in marijuana regulation. And there is always the Supreme Court with their infinite wisdom to rule on every imaginable marijuana challenge that will inevitably develop.

On the state level we have their own bicameral legislatures to contend with. Then there is their Departments of Health, Departments of Revenue, and their Alcohol and Tobacco Control Boards, and of course all of their various court Levels.

Most important, at *every* level, federal and state, and aimed at every gullible (at best) and vulnerable individual in every agency at every step along the way, **we have the special interest lobbyists muddying the waters with their endless perks and cash**.

We now have forty jurisdictions that have managed to pass some sort of pro-marijuana legislation. The federal government has, at least to date, taken themselves out of the equation and allowed the states to decide whether *Marijuana – The Wonder Weed* should be banned, allowed for medical use, or allowed for full recreational use.

Washington, Oregon, Colorado, Alaska and The District of Columbia have decided: "YES TO ALL USES". Score a few biggies for our side! Expect more in November 2016.

Florida tried, but by requiring a 60% "super-majority" and not a simple 50% majority vote their effort fell a scant 2% short with 58% voting "YES". Florida, along with a handful of other states with similar votes in the offing should see legalization soon on either the medical, recreational, or on both levels.

In many now-legal states the legislatures passed bills allowing

49

some strictly- limited medical use of marijuana and its derivatives. Each state is quite different. Some strongly restrict the number of dispensary licenses. Some allow users to grow their own plants. Many do not. Some restrict the physical ingestion to "vaping only" or "edibles only".

Other states allow use for a wide variety of illnesses. The taxing structures differ widely. There is absolutely NO universal agreement on *any* matter you can think of. Not even close.

Is actually achieving voter or legislative approval the end of any battle for legalization? Far from it! It is only a start. Colorado and Oregon are the "petri dishes", the lab experiments if you will, for full legalization. Here is where the turf battles have come into play and become evident.

Who regulates what? Who controls what? Who gets their pound of flesh? How do you price legal marijuana to discourage the black market? How do you prevent under-age use? How do you decide if a driver is impaired? How do you keep the cartels out of the grow-plots? These are all very legitimate and thorny concerns to address.

This is a **_very_** complex issue. Regulators try to control land use, growing methods, strain limitations, seed-to-sale tracking by each *individual* seed (!), shipping, packaging, wholesaling, retailing, personnel at every level, policing and pricing.

Even *where* one is permitted to physically be located to consume marijuana is an issue. So are in what *form* can one ingest marijuana, how much marijuana and derivative products one can *buy* in a given time frame, and how much one can have on their person. These are all tightly regulated.

You name it, someone in some group, usually more than one

group, wants to define the parameters. No one wants to cede even a small amount of their authority. Turf wars!

As a strong believer in States' Rights I do think the federal government should pass final legislation totally decriminalizing marijuana, un-scheduling or re-scheduling to Schedule III, and leaving it up to the voters in *each state* to decide on matters of decriminalization and level of availability.

From that point on one can best argue that the states should simply learn as they go (think Colorado, Oregon and Washington) and eventually everything will work itself out. In our Constitutional Republic it somehow usually does.

The entire issue of the Legalization of Marijuana is a shining example of American democracy and American entrepreneurship at its finest. May GOD, who put the healing herbal plant marijuana on this earth, eternally bless America.

The battle for marijuana legalization must take its place among the litany of threats and problems we puny humans face on a daily basis. Where it fits in the list of "life's problems and dangers" can be debated endlessly. The fact is that many of these daily problems are *far* beyond the scope of what any individual or even any *nation* could possibly influence. The legalization of marijuana is **not** one of them.

For the super-paranoid, this list could be very scary. For the well informed, it is just a compilation of threats from the **improbable** to the **foreseeable** to the **ever-present**. Consider the following:

The **improbable**, over which we all have zero control:

- Threats from beyond our solar system. These could Include hostile alien invasion (really?), or huge bursts of radiation from exploding galaxies (which do exist).

- Threats from beyond our planet but within our solar system. These include direct hits from comets and asteroids (which snuffed out the dinosaurs), and solar flares (which totally fried our infant electrical grid about 150 years ago and could be more devastating today.)

The **foreseeable**, over which we have limited control as a nation:

- A surprise nuclear attack. (Remember Pearl Harbor?)
- A cyber-attack permanently shutting down our power grid. (Possibly our single greatest threat as a nation.)
- An attack by ISIS on American soil. (Got any idea where all those missing suitcase nukes are?)
- A monetary collapse worldwide.

The **ever-present**, over which we have various levels of control, *if we have the will*:

- Wars on foreign soils.
- Climate Change, man-made or otherwise.
    (SPACE LEFT HERE INTENTIONALLY)
- *Unemployment and underemployment.*
- *Poverty.*
- *Racial unrest.*
- *Addiction to alcohol and tobacco.*
- *Chronic obesity.*
- *Prescription drug addiction.*
- *Street drug addiction.*
- *Severe illnesses, cancer, HIV, and dozens more.*

I'm sure I've missed a few, but the above list gives me enough chills!

Here is why I mention these potential threats and problems in this book. The last eight in the above list, below the open space, of the "ever-present" problems, could be reduced to a greater or lesser extent **by legalizing marijuana!**

I hope to show throughout this book why this statement is difficult to refute.

CHAPTER 6
BIG PHARMA = BIG PROBLEM

Deborah Norville, Emmy Award-Winning TV Personality: "I think it's great... They're gonna regulate marijuana the way alcohol is regulated. People are smoking it and doing it anyway. In the state of Washington they figured out you're gonna save half a billion dollars in revenues from the taxes that this will generate. And think of what you're not spending in terms of the law enforcement that's frankly being wasted on people who are doing it in the privacy of their own home."

Throughout this book I pick on "Big Pharma", the massive multi-national drug companies. I do this because **THEY** are in fact the #1 enemy today in the fight for legalization of marijuana. Here's why:

A study done in 2015 that was published in *The Annual Review of Public Health* showed some amazing statistics:

- Total annual sales of 72 kilograms (158 pounds) of pain killers per 100,000 people (a mere <u>276 tons</u>; that's a hell of a lot of little white pills);

- Deaths from overdoses were an astounding 54 per 100,000 people (over 189,000 individuals, an average of 500+ per day);

- Hospital admissions for overdoses was an amazing 410 per 100,000 people (over a million and a quarter (1,435,000) individuals! This is an average of over 3,900 overdoses daily.)

This qualifies as a massive **EPEDEMIC**!

The *key* Big Pharma opioid product we are talking about here is OxyContin, generically oxycodone hydrochloride.

It all began about twenty years ago when, in the mid '90s Big Pharma literally brainwashed doctors into prescribing OxyContin for pain relief. Statistically almost one in three Americans suffers from some form of chronic pain, so the potential profit for the pharmaceutical industry was enormous.

It is reported that during the six years after 1996 Purdue Pharmaceutical alone funded over 20,000 "scientific" papers! These were all focused on convincing doctors to prescribe opioid painkillers for chronic pain.

Purdue poured millions of dollars of contributions (bribes?) into the waiting arms of The American Pain Society, The American Academy of Pain Medicine, The Federation of State Medical Boards and The Joint Commission on Drugs, and many others. In return for the "donations" these groups all advocated strongly for the use of the new wonder-opioids.

The studies themselves made highly misleading claims, backed by nothing but pure hype. They asserted that OxyContin and related painkillers were safer than all other available pain medications. **They knew otherwise**.

Eventually, after countless deaths, the government woke up and fined Purdue $634,000,000 for their misleading information, as reported by the Associated Press in 2007.

But inertia is unstoppable. This was a drop in the bucket compared to opioid profits. Millions of Americans were *already* addicted to OyxContin. In 2012 alone over 300,000,000 (three hundred million!) opioid prescriptions were written. Result: 47,000 opioid-related overdose deaths in the

United States alone. This has grown yearly, and was reported to be over 50,000 in 2015.

What is wrong? How can this possibly be allowed to continue? Nixon's **"WAR ON DRUGS"**, that's what is wrong.

Fueled by the "hippie" counter-cultural movement of the '60s Richard Nixon's failed (in his viewpoint) marijuana study (see Chapter 3) was tossed in the trash can. He famously stated: "If we cannot destroy the drug menace in America then it will surely in time destroy us."

Nixon initiated his massive global escalation of police and military actions. These efforts resulted in mass incarcerations in the United States (mostly black youths) proliferation of drug-related violence worldwide, destruction of minority communities, and the escalation of cartel violence mostly related to heroin. Thanks Tricky Dick!

America alone has spent to date over $1,000,000,000,000 (that's one trillion dollars!) on the War On Drugs. It has been an abysmal failure.

It is reported that since 2009 the FDA has collected over $2,500,000,000 ($2.5 Billion!) in **kickbacks from Big Pharma**! This was for the favors of rapidly approving ("fast-tracking") extremely dangerous opioid drugs. These blatant bribes clearly also were intended to prevent, or at least delay, the legalization of marijuana.

The American Medical Association has reported that over 106,000 people die EVERY YEAR from Food and Drug Administration *approved* drugs after being USED AS DIRECTED.

There are two reasons why Big Pharma is terrified of the legalization of marijuana:

- Marijuana has the potential to replace all opioid pain killers, and *many* other prescription drugs;

- When they do produce their own marijuana-based, or even a synthetic marijuana, as prescription meds, they cannot begin to compete in the open market with the authentic Wonder Weed in price or effectiveness.

Regarding opioids, Big Pharma produces 276 tons (!) yearly. The VA hospitals are perhaps their largest client. Opioids are highly addictive. They kill thousands yearly from overdoses intended or otherwise. (Think Prince.) They do control pain, but also cause extreme constipation.

But wait! Of course Big Pharma has the answer to that as well. Enter "OID", advertised extensively to relieve constipation caused by their own opioids! What a sweet business model! Make money causing a problem. Make additional money resolving the problem you caused! Sweet.

Here's their concern. The primary benefit of marijuana, among its countless other medicinal benefits, is its ability to relieve pain. It is non-addictive, and not one person in history of the world has ever died from an overdose. Sufficient reason for Big Pharma's bottom-line concern? You betcha!

GW Pharmaceuticals in England has produced a tincture from plants at their own rather secretive marijuana farm. I saw a video about this on TV recently, one bit of a three-part six-hour documentary. They have created "SATAVIX".

As an MS patient myself I have searched for years for relief from the excruciating pain and debilitating spasms that manifests my personal form of MS. To date only cannabidiol (CBD) offers me proven relief.

I read about the successes MS patients apparently had using Satavix. As far as I could determine it was available only in Canada and New Zealand. (Of course it had not yet been approved in the United States.) Here's the rub:

The cost for SATAVIX hovers around two hundred dollars for a ten milliliter vial! At the prescribed dose it equates to around $7,000.00/year! This, incidentally, is about a half-billion dollars a year if every MS patient in the UK alone were to use it! No wonder Big Pharma is pouring untold millions of dollars to lobby politicians to insure that Harry Anslinger's dream of marijuana prohibition in the United States lives on forever.

Well, OK. If I were rich SATAVIX might well be worth it. Or, if at some time in the future, some health care plan might actually cover most or all of the expense, great. BUT, here is where Big Pharma is terrified. That same ten milliliters of concentrated cannabis oil could be produced privately, according to published guidelines, for **under ten bucks**! That's one twentieth, five percent, of GW's selling price! Wow!

What is even more extraordinary is that CBD rich hemp oil can today be bought over the counter legally anywhere in the United States! Until recently all hemp oil had to be produced outside of the United States and imported. This was because our uninformed politicians thought hemp and Schedule I marijuana were exactly the same thing. They *sound* the same. They are *not* the same. (See Chapters 10 and 12)

It is only within the past two years that the federal government is allowing states to begin hemp growing programs. Big Pharma lost this round. Hemp prohibition began when marijuana was victimized in 1937.

The government mandated that hemp growing be resuscitated for four years during the WWII war effort. The ban was reapplied shortly after the war ended. It took another *sixty years* for sanity to begin to prevail.

Getting back to opioid pain killers, those most commonly prescribed are:

- HYDROCODONE (Vicodin)
- HYDROMORPHONE (Dilaudid)
- MEPERIDINE (Demerol)
- METHODONE (Dolophine)
- MORPHINE (Roxanol; morphine sulfate)
- OXYCODONE (Percocet; OxyContin) The #1 prescribed opioid.
- OXYMORPHONE (Opana) From Endo Pharm
- FENTANYL --- R.I.P. Prince.

Fentanyl is a Schedule II drug, thereby considered by Uncle Sam to be **safer** than harmless marijuana! It is BY FAR the most powerful and deadly opioid ever created. It is extremely easy to overdose. A SINGLE GRAM, a small amount of powder, is said to be able to supply 7,000 pain-killing doses!

Fentanyl is eighty to one-hundred *TIMES* as powerful as morphine. It was created to mitigate extreme post-operative pain, and is seldom prescribed for any other reason. How did Prince obtain a fatal dose? Was he ever told just how dangerous a substance this opioid is? We may never know.

Minnesota, where Prince resided, is one of the states where medical marijuana is legal. Why was Prince never prescribed marijuana for his problems? We may never know that either.

Legally-prescribed opioids are a serious epidemic. But it brings in around $9,000,000,000 (nine billion dollars!) to Big Pharmas' coffers. No wonder they are terrified of marijuana legalization!

Please read Chapter 24 for a more in-depth study of the killer drugs that Big Pharma has managed to get *fast tracked* and judged to be safe. This was entirely irrespective of whether they can kill! **This is one of America's greatest scandals.**

In June 2015 Time Magazine reported that of the 9,400,000 Americans who take opioids for long term pain, the National Institute of Health estimates that 2,100,000 are firmly addicted. <u>Four out of five heroin addicts say they came to heroin through opioids.</u> Prescription opioids are <u>by far</u> the #1 gateway drug in America.

A reported average of 46 Americans die every day from prescribed opioid overdoses. For middle-aged citizens a prescription opioid overdose is a more likely cause of death than an auto accident or a violent crime.

Weak research opened up the door to opioid overuse. The corrupt Food and Drug Administration approved ever more powerful drugs for long-term use based **ONLY** on studies of their *short term* use and efficacy. The reasoning was that long term studies could not be conducted because the placebo control group would be needlessly subjected to unrelieved pain. Now there is classic government head-up-the-ass reasoning! I wonder who dictated THAT thinking?

In early 2016 the government in its infinite wisdom issued new physician guidelines "imploring" physicians to prescribe fewer opioid pain killers. This will inevitably lead to those in chronic pain buying contaminated opioids on the street. The black market in opioids is thriving in every major city in the United States. (See Chapter 23 regarding street drugs).

An estimated 100,000,000 Americans suffer from chronic pain. This is about one in three of our citizens. The Institute of Medicine reports that a quarter of these, 25,000,000, say the pain is severe enough to affect their day to day activities. THIS defines Big Pharmas' huge market. THIS is why cannabinoid medicines, which are non-addictive and CANNOT KILL, **must** be legalized.

Of course drug companies have been scrambling to produce a "substitute marijuana". They came up with "Marinol", which the government promptly granted <u>Schedule III status</u>! Let's see.....REAL marijuana is Schedule I; Big Pharma's substitute marijuana is Schedule III. <u>What an amazing coincidence!</u>

The FDA approval process focuses on a **single drug/single target** approach. This very conveniently sidesteps approving marijuana. As the FDA puts it: "The problem is in dealing with the complexities and interactions of whole plant medicines such as marijuana. Herbal cannabis has many different active ingredients targeting multiple targets in the body." Duh! That's why and how marijuana actually works its medical magic!

THAT'S THE POINT YOU BUFFOONS! It is the synergy between all of those "complexities" that makes marijuana the magical herbal medicine that has been recognized as such for centuries! Big Pharma knows it and wishes the public didn't. **<u>WAKE UP AMERICA</u>!**

Studies conducted with Big Pharma's Marinol vs herbal marijuana have demonstrated far fewer side effects using natural herbal marijuana. Further, with vaporized marijuana accurate doses are far easier to achieve than with oral Marinol. The most important fact is that marijuana contains dozens of medically-useful <u>synergistic components</u> that are entirely missing from Marinol.

WHY IS IT THAT *FOUR* PRESTIGIOUS <u>HOSPITALS</u> IN ISRAEL HAVE ALREADY INSTALLED MARIJUANA

VAPORIZORS PERMANENTLY FOR THEIR PATIENTS USE? <u>BECAUSE IT WORKS!</u> *WAKE UP AMERICA!*

The fact is that no matter how hard Big Pharma tries to produc a substitute marijuana they are doomed to failure.

As mentioned above, GW Pharmaceuticals in England produce a concentrated marijuana oil spray called Sativex. It is not a synthetic. It has been fully approved for use throughout Europe, and in Canada and New Zealand. It is apparently also undergoing United States trials.

Sativex is intended primarily to treat multiple sclerosis spasticity, neuropathic pain, and cancer pain. It is a spray that delivers 2.7mg THC and 2.5mg CBD directly into the mouth. As I said earlier, Satavix is extremely expensive. There are, however, instructions in *The Medicinal Cannabis Guidebook* by Jeff Ditchfield et al for producing a superior product for under $10.00!

Of course, if GW Pharma is ever granted United States patent protection, as they are attempting to achieve, "homemade Satavix" will be as illegal as home grown marijuana.

Since I'm picking on Big Pharma anyway why not bring up an interesting "conspiracy theory" for those so inclined. (Skip the following few paragraphs if you are offended by conspiracy theories!)

Nagalese is a toxic protein found in high levels in cancer patients and autistic children. There exists a very effective antidote, GcMAF, another protein. It is effectively used in Europe, but as with many other drugs that have been proven to be effective in patients overseas, it is illegal in the United States. Even so, a number of fearless American doctors have successfully cured patients using GcMAF.

These doctors disclosed that they believed that Nagalese

62

was being <u>INTENTIONALLY</u> added to vaccines by Big Pharma! And guess what? These doctors unexpectedly either died or disappeared without a trace!

The most famous of these cases was that of eminent autism researcher Dr. Bradstreet. Three days before his body was found in a river with a bullet hole in his head his office was ransacked and all of his research papers were stolen.

After a leading CDC (Center for Disease Control) scientist admitted that the CDC had destroyed documents outlining the direct relationship between the MMR vaccine (mumps, measles, rubella) and autism in black kids, Rep. Bill Posey (R-FL) on July 29, 2015 called for a full Congressional investigation. The request fell on deaf ears. The influence of Big Pharma on our politicians is *huge*. **Believe it.**

Can you REALLY blame Big Pharma for caring more about profits than about patients? This is the epitome of American Capitalism, is it not?

Picture yourself an executive of a big pharmaceutical company. The company's stock is traded on a major public stock exchange. The company is supposed to "answer to" its thousands of investors and show a consistent profit. It might even generously share some of these with investors as dividends. The company employs thousands, if not tens of thousands of employees who depend upon it for their very survival.

This same company has spent untold millions of dollars in research to create complex chemical formulations that may relieve or even cure a vast range of medical conditions.

Now imagine if someone, perhaps a medical professional but probably not, comes along and says: "Wait a minute big shot executive, virtually everything you produce can have serious side effects, ***including death***, as *you yourself* acknowledge in small print in the flyer included with every prescription." "In addition, you produce deadly opioids that have a big percentage of Americans hooked for life. You are killing us off at a rapid clip, and killing our PTSD afflicted vets even faster. **Well, I've got something that is much safer that could very well put you out of business!"**

"My product is a simple natural herbal plant, essentially a weed. It has been studied and used effectively for thousands of years. Your killer chemicals have been scarcely studied at all, each for a few years at best. Further, my product is far safer, less expensive, and as effective or better than your chemical concoctions..... **AND WE HAVE COUNTLESS STUDIES TO PROVE IT!"**

As such an executive, don't you think you might be at least *mildly* concerned? How about in a ***total panic***? This is the worried state of the pharmaceutical industry today as it is faced with the eventual inevitability of universal legalization of marijuana. Profits speak louder than compassion.

Big Pharma plows untold billions of dollars into advertising and perks directed at the American Medical Association (AMA) and every physician on the planet! Further, they employ lobbyists that pretty much "own" the political establishment. Money talks, logic and truth often sadly walks.

How else can one possibly explain the misinformation that has been presented to the public through the media for decades? How else can one explain why *very few* physicians, even in states where marijuana has been legalized, will prescribe it for any reason? In my state of Arizona I have yet to find ONE.

How can one POSSIBLY explain why our federal government classifies marijuana as a Schedule I controlled substance

Alongside deadly addictive crack cocaine and heroin, while Big Pharma gets a pass time after time after time?

I'll tell you how: **Big Pharma**, and its bottomless chest of funds to promote their agenda and bribe every politician and doctor in sight, that's how! Can you blame them? If you believe that corporate profits are more important than public health, than you simply *cannot* blame them.

If you believe that the pain and suffering of millions alive today and in the future should count more than Big Pharmas' bottom line, please join us in every way you can to help get marijuana decriminalized and legalized across America.

One way any American can help this cause is to donate any amount no matter how small to one or more of the non-profit legalization advocate organizations listed in Appendix II. Please consider our own Arizona non-profit group: The National Weed Legalization Fund at TNWLF.org.

Thank you in advance for your help!

CHAPTER 7
ENDLESS BAD PRESS

HOW THE MEDIA HURTS MARIJUNA LEGALIZATION EFFORTS

Alan Colmes, Host of Fox News Radio's "Alan Colmes Show":
"No matter what else is going on in the world, whenever we do a marijuana topic we get a huge reaction. I think most Americans have a very libertarian view about this... The government should stay out of it, not make it illegal, sell it like any other substance, tax it... You talk about ways to solve our budget problem -- legalize drugs, legalize marijuana."

Mark Twain (Samuel Clemens), Author:
"It's very easy to fool the people, but very hard to un-fool them."

There is absolutely no question that Mark Twain was entirely correct. The American public has been "fooled", lied to endlessly for eighty years, about the imagined "evils" of marijuana. Only in the past decade has any progress been made "un-fooling" Americans.

Marijuana has been used as medicine and for religious purposes for over 5,000 years. It has been unearthed in ancient Chinese tombs and in vessels from bronze-age Scythia. An ancient Chinese doctor created a complete written pharmacopeia.

Texts from ancient India describe a wide range of medicinal benefits. Its use as a valued medicine and in religious ceremonies has been documented for centuries throughout Africa and the Middle East.

So what happened to demonize a natural medicinal healing herb that was such a popular and widely used medicine for centuries? Sadly, a lot of lies have happened. The media is mostly responsible for perpetuating these lies to this day.

Hemp, a variant of the same plant as marijuana, came to America on the Mayflower! Our early colonists were actually mandated by law to grow hemp, a very useful raw material. George Washington and Thomas Jefferson grew it. At one time taxes could be paid in hemp! Most early American paper was made from hemp fiber, including the paper used to write The Declaration of Independence! (For more information on hemp see Chapter 12.)

The more psychoactive variants of cannabis, Indica and Sativa marijuana, used worldwide for millennia, eventually became popular in America among writers, artists and musicians. They were convinced that its psychoactive influence greatly enhanced their creativity.

A book written in 1857 by an author named Fitz Lodlow titled *The Hasheesh Eater* (actually his autobiography) introduced many of the readers of the day to the wonders of recreational marijuana use.

Throughout the following decades musicians in particular found that using marijuana helped them hear notes better and actually play better.

Keep in mind, the late 1800s and early 1900s were the days when "opium dens" were vilified as dens of iniquity, and Coca Cola actually contained *real* cocaine!

Enter the mass-media newspapers of the day. They recognized that sensational coverage of *anything* sold papers. Recreational drugs qualified. Vilifying them with totally fabricated articles sold lots of papers. In 1926 The New Orleans Morning Tribune ran a series of extremely misleading articles on the "growing menace of cannabis". Just to sell papers! Imagine that. Shocking? Not really.

Other newspapers caught on to the idea, and managed to inject the race angle into the anti-marijuana rhetoric. They linked "black madness and mayhem" to their use of marijuana supposedly far in excess of white persons' used. **It was a total lie.**

Just to sell papers, fictitious scare stories with headlines such as: "Marijuana causes white women to seek relations with Negroes", and "Teen slaughters family with axe after smoking marijuana" were published. The gullible public soaked it all up like a dry sponge.

A few states, initially Massachusetts, passed inane laws outlawing this terrible public menace. Overseas, an anti-marijuana speech by an Egyptian delegate to an international drug conference, wherein he compared marijuana to the hated opium, led to England outlawing marijuana in 1928. They beat us to it!

Perhaps the single event that most shaped public opinion about marijuana was the idiotic 1936 movie "*Reefer Madness*". This Grade C- flick, horribly written and even worse acted, actually was a *big* part of the impetus for the first anti-marijuana law ever enacted in the United States.

Incidentally, you can buy modern DVDs of *Reefer Madness* on line. It is so ridiculous that it is actually hilarious when viewed with our present understanding of marijuana. Wellworth the price.

Furious over Anslinger's vilification of "marihuana", which of course he knew was actually the popular medicine cannabis, was a brave Dr. William Woodward. He represented the American Medical Association.

Woodward argued *vehemently* before Congress: "I say the medicinal use of cannabis has absolutely nothing to do with addiction. Further investigation will show that there are substantial medical uses for cannabis."

In spite of Woodward's passionate testimony, in 1937 the United States Congress passed Harry Anslinger's "Marihuana Tax Act" making anything "cannabis" illegal nationwide for any purpose as it is to this day.

The wealthy complicit newspaper magnate William Randolph Hearst published, for reasons of his own, all of Harry Anslinger's racist anti-black anti-Mexican anti-marijuana lies. **ALL of the articles were pure fiction!** They fooled the American public, and it has taken the better part of a century to even begin to un-fool them.

Twenty-four years after the United States made marijuana illegal, one-hundred-eighty countries signed the "United Nations Single Convention On Narcotic Drugs", including marijuana. This brought the rest of the world in line with American prohibition of marijuana for any purpose whatsoever. (Four other nations signed on later.)

This document was crafted by none other than the American Bureau of Narcotics Director Harry Anslinger. It was essentially an updating of a 1931 Paris Convention on drugs which had NOT included marijuana.

What came next was the final crushing blow. Because of the

increasing popularity and use of marijuana despite its illegal status, President Nixon created the Shafer Commission to study the "Devil's Weed" and prove to America that prohibition was the correct path to follow forever. He apparently had pre-conceived notions about the outcome! The results of this fiasco were discussed earlier, leading to the War On Drugs.

What I find most distressing are little subtleties buried in articles that we see every day on the internet and in the media. These statements are heard so often they have become "givens", never challenged or researched by anyone as being factual.

Here is one example from a Motley Fool (Their Motto: "To Educate, Amuse, Enrich") article on 6/22/15. I was *not* amused (nor surprised) to read that: "Researchers have decades' worth of studies focused on the dangers of marijuana to sift through with a corresponding ***snippet*** of data concerning the benefits of marijuana use." (Emphasis mine.)

SNIPPET??? There are 5,000+ years-worth of data on the many benefits of the Wonder Weed marijuana to "sift through". Literally *countless* volumes of anecdotal testimony exists from users who derive real-life medical benefits from ingesting marijuana to successfully treat a wide variety of ailments.

Then there merely the hundreds of real scientific studies, many done by the federal government itself! To refer to this irrefutable huge body of anecdotal and scientific evidence as a "*snippet* of data" is simply ludicrous and *intentionally* grossly misleading.

There is a subtle bias in media reporting almost every day. For example, there are literally hundreds of Big Pharmas' drug-related opioid deaths in the United States every week. They are *never* reported. BUT, as with the April 2016 Ohio

70

killings, they made headlines for weeks because **marijuana** grow facilities, *unrelated* to the crime, were supposedly found at the *location* of the crime. If they had found a meth lab it would not have made page C5.

Because Colorado is the "petri dish" study of full legalization, reports of their progress are appearing in the media that are extremely misleading. This is how the media distorts reality:

REPORT: "Arrests in Colorado for driving under the influence of marijuana skyrocket!" Well, duh! If they weren't even testing for marijuana influence a year ago, if there is one single arrest, the number is up a staggering 100%! Just plain nuts.

REPORT: "Emergency rooms see huge increase in marijuana overdoses!" This one is almost funny. First off, when anyone thinks of a hospital emergency room they think of a person near death from a stroke or heart attack, or bleeding to death from a gunshot or stab wound, or near death from an overdose of a legal prescription medicine.

Persons admitted for a marijuana overdose are not near death…NO ONE HAS EVER DIED FROM A MARIJUANA OVERDOSE. NO ONE EVER WILL!

For the most part these folks are just scared to death and sleepy as hell! They experienced an effect they didn't expect and never before felt. Obviously time for a 911 call!

I have not seen any study of how many of these "marijuana emergencies" were from first time users. I will bet it is a *very* high percentage. The first time someone smokes a joint, or eats a marijuana-laced brownie, they have absolutely no idea what to expect. The "high" that is experienced the first time, if sufficiently intense, can be truly frightening. Not at all unpleasant, just frightening!

71

I can relate! It happened to me with my first marijuana dark chocolate bar. I did not heed the warning on the label: "Ingest tiny bites until you are comfortable with the effect, which can take hours." I ate the whole damn delicious bar in about thirty seconds! Yummm.

Next thing I knew I struggling to get to the phone, which was about two feet away from the bed! I had to call my wife to tell her to get someone to drive her home from work because I was paralyzed! Happy, but paralyzed. It passed in a few hours. Emergency? Far from it. I can certainly relate to someone thinking a 911 call and a visit to the ER was a life-or-death necessity!

Another misrepresentation that appears all too frequently in the media is when they refer to kids overdosing on a common street-drug known as "Spice" or "Moon Rocks". The media insists on referring to Spice overdoses as "an overdose of *synthetic marijuana*". Heck, if they can die from the *synthetic* stuff the REAL stuff must be REALLY bad. Obvious conclusion. Just totally wrong.

Fact: <u>There is zero, absolute zero, chemical resemblance between what the media insists in calling "synthetic marijuana",</u> Spice, and the wonderful healing herbal medicine marijuana. One kills. The other cures.

Slowly and painfully the battle for legalization of marijuana and its many derivative products is being won across America. Because of the overwhelming positive evidence of marijuana's value it becomes simply a matter of **educating the public, effectively un-fooling them.** Education will allow the wonderful process of democracy to take its course.

72

It is a shameful, criminal situation, that so many people need to continue to suffer needlessly while the legalization process very slowly unfolds and our federal government watches in mute uncaring silence.

Shame on our government.

CHAPTER 8
THE PHENOMONON
OF THE "FIRST NEWS"

George Soros, Chairman of Soros Fund Management:
"Who most benefits from keeping marijuana illegal? The greatest beneficiaries are the major criminal organizations in Mexico and elsewhere that earn billions of dollars annually from this illicit trade--and who would rapidly lose their competitive advantage if marijuana were a legal commodity. Some claim that they would only move into other illicit enterprises, but they are more likely to be weakened by being deprived of the easy profits they can earn with marijuana."

No one can deny we live in the "Information Age". Until the internet became commonplace, news spread more slowly. Even in the recent 1980's radio and TV were far slower than cyberspace and the internet. But one fact has always been true: THE NEWS THAT IS <u>FIRST REPORTED</u> IS THE NEWS THAT IS <u>LONGEST REMEMBERED</u>.

Later retractions, even full refutations of the original "news", are often relegated to the back pages and are never again headline news. **First impressions count.**

A perfect example is the Ferguson, Missouri tragic shooting of an unarmed (albeit criminal) teenager. "Hands Up...Don't Shoot", the victim's alleged last words before being gunned down by a "rotten" cop. These words have forever been implanted in the psyche of a large segment of the U.S. population. They are accepted as irrefutable "fact".

The *true* fact is that the far-lesser-reported *eye-witness accounts* later proved **beyond any doubt** that those words were **never** spoken. This can **NEVER** undo the original headlines. The rotten white cop in Ferguson shot a defenseless black kid who was trying his best to surrender. "Hands up".....:"Don't shoot!" **First impressions count.**

I won't even get into our government's monthly glowingly-positive "FIRST NEWS" "financial numbers reports" that are INVARIABLY revised to their correct <u>less-favorable</u> figures the following month! Don't we EVER get the message? First impressions count, and the government uses it continuously to its benefit.

So it is with marijuana. I can recall vividly a sensational story I heard back in the early '80s which until recently I kept in my memory bank as a possible negative to my interest in legalization of marijuana. Could I *possibly* be wrong? I should have known better!

On September 28, 1980 the Washington Post began a series of featured articles by a reporter named Janet Cooke. The articles chronicled the sad and horrific life of a little eight-year-old boy named "Jimmy". He lived in a squalid drug-user house where marijuana smoking was rampant. Jimmy himself had become an addict. Poor, poor drugged-out little Jimmy.

These featured articles raised national outrage. Every anti-marijuana organization in the country seized the opportunity to jump on the bandwagon. The series was discussed in newspapers everywhere. Janet Cooke became a national hero for her brave reporting.

The series was so powerful and compelling that on April 13, 1981 Janet Cook received writing's most prestigious award for her "brave reporting"….**The Pulitzer Prize**!

Her noble and brilliant reporting once and for all documented the "known" evils of the Devil's-Weed and other drugs, and she had been aptly rewarded. Jimmy's was a truly heart wrenching account, quite *worthy* of a Pulitzer Prize. It made anyone who ever questioned the evils of marijuana to think twice about their obviously wrong feelings.

Shortly thereafter health authorities and school officials tried to locate poor little Jimmy to remove him from his drug-plagued existence. **Shockingly, they couldn't find him. Anywhere! Where was poor little Jimmy? Where?**

Guess what? Under intense pressure and questioning Janet Cooke finally admitted **THE ENTIRE STORY WAS A FABRICATION! IT WAS 100% FICTION! MS. COOK MADE IT *ALL* UP! THERE WAS NO "POOR LITTLE JIMMY". THE PULITZER PRIZE COMMITTEE TOOK BACK HER PULITZER PRIZE THE VERY NEXT DAY!**

Once again, the "evil-marijuana" agenda seed had been nurtured nationwide. (Let's not forget that ridiculous '30s anti-marijuana movie "Reefer Madness".) Marijuana was "in fact" a great evil. Some poor kid's experience conclusively proved it.

Even worse, had the story in the Washington Post series actually been acknowledged as **_untrue_**, many would conclude: "So what? *Surely* some other poor kid somewhere was going through the exact same situation." The public never forgot the story of "Poor Little Jimmy". I remember it to this day. **First impressions count.**

CHAPTER 9
FEDERAL DRUG SCHEDULES

Paul McCartney, Beatles Lead Singer, Composer:
"I support decriminalization. People are smoking pot anyway and to make them into criminals is wrong. It's when you're in jail you really become a criminal."

The United States passed the "Controlled Substances Act" in 1937. Under this act there are five categories, or "Schedules", under which controlled substances are categorized.

It is important to understand the *two* underlying features of *each* of the five Schedules, because **this is what is at the heart of the entire marijuana legalization issue:**

1. Medical value is based ONLY on long-term large-scale controlled clinical trials. These are the so-called replicable "double blind clinical studies" performed in government certified laboratories by credentialed physicians, and subject to peer review.

2. "Potential for abuse" is based on the relative likelihood that an individual will take a substance ON THEIR OWN INITIATIVE (i.e., without a prescription) leading to personal health hazards and public endangerment.

ONLY Schedule I drugs are considered to have NO MEDICAL VALUE, "1" above. Potential for abuse, "2", is for all intents and purposes, irrelevant for marijuana because "1" is virtually impossible to accomplish with the almost limitless marijuana strains and variants. "2" will never come into play.

Schedule II drugs can have extremely high potential for abuse

("2"), but have shown "some", however small, medical value ("1"). Think fentanyl.

Schedule III, IV and V drugs have varying degrees of medical value and abuse potential.

Restated:

SCHEDULE I:

- No accepted medical use.
- No accepted safety standard for use under medical supervision.

  Examples: heroin, LSD, peyote (mescaline), Quaaludes (methaqualone), ecstasy (3,4,methylene dioxy methamphetamine), crack cocaine, **marijuana.**

SCHEDULE II:

- Proven medicinal value.
- High potential for abuse

  Examples: dilaudid, morphene, codeine, oxycontin, Percocet, opium, Demerol, amobarbitol, pentobarbital, Ritalin, desoxyn (methamphetamine), amphisome (dexadrone), Adderall, fentanyl.

SCHEDULE III:

- Proven medicinal value.
- Moderate potential for abuse

  Examples: **Marinol;** Vicodin (under 15mg/dose), Tylenol w/codeine (under 90mg codeine/dose), didrex, ketamine, anabolic steroids, testosterone.

Marinol, Big Pharma's "marijuana substitute" was

apparently *magically* judged to have accepted medical use and accepted safety standards. What a surprise!

SCHEDULE IV:

- Proven medical value.
- Low potential for abuse.

   Examples: xanex, sona, klonopin, tranxene, valium, ativan, temezapam, halcion.

SCHEDULE V:

- Proven medical value.
- No abuse potential.

   Examples: aspirin and similar over-the counter products, cough medicines with minimal codeine.

Marijuana is **SCHEDULE I FOR ONE AND ONLY ONE REASON:** The United States government defiantly refuses to accept the fact that marijuana could have even the **slightest** medical value! **How utterly absurd is that?**

Incidentally: Schedule I crack cocaine (the same Schedule as marijuana) today is considered the biggest drug threat by far in the United States.

Throughout this book I pick on "Big Pharma", the massive multi-national drug companies, because **THEY** are the #1 enemy in the fight for legalization of marijuana. Here's why:

A study done in 2015 that was published in *The Annual Review of Public Health* showed some amazing statistics:

- Total sales of 72 kilograms (158 pounds) of pain killers per 100,000 people (Based on our population of 350 million, this is a mere 276 tons; that's a hell of a lot of little white pain-killing pills!

- Deaths from overdoses were an astounding 54 per 100,000 people (over 189,000 individuals, an average of 550 per day!)

- Hospital admissions for overdoses was an amazing 410 per 100,000 people (That's almost a million and a half [1,435,000] individuals!) This is an average of almost 4,000 overdoses daily!

This qualifies as a massive **EPEDEMIC**! It also qualifies as **huge** profits for Big Pharma. Surprise!

Remember, we are talking here about Schedule II classified LEGAL drugs! The primary key Big Pharma opioid product we are talking about here is OxyContin, generically oxycodone hydrochloride.

It all began about twenty years ago when, in the mid '90s, Big Pharma literally *brainwashed* doctors into prescribing OxyContin for pain relief. Statistically almost one in three Americans suffers from some form of chronic pain, so the potential profit for the pharmaceutical industry was enormous!

NOTE: Schedule II drugs are the opioids (think OxyContin), and methamphetamines! Irrespective of their highly addictive properties ("2") and the FACT that hundreds of thousands have died from overdoses (versus **ZERO** deaths from marijuana overdoses), "scientific studies" of opioids, such as those by Purdue Pharma back in the '90s, apparently showed SOME medical benefit.

The severity of criminal penalties for drug possession, sale and use follow the above Schedules, generally speaking. BUT, as with marijuana, states can make their own modifications to the federal drug laws, though always under the threat of federal enforcement.

Even the feds modify their insane laws on occasion. In the mid-'80s, in response to a growing epidemic of crack cocaine use, criminal penalties were increased to Schedule I levels.

Here some food for thought: <u>In 1970, under intense lobbying pressure (money talks, logic walks!) alcohol, tobacco and caffeine, (booze and smokes and coffee **clearly SCHEDULE I** under the above definitions), were *specifically exempted* from Scheduling!</u>

Of course, the immense human suffering and loss of life from both alcohol and tobacco is irrefutably well documented.

Clearly, given sufficient reason, Schedules *can* be changed. Why not marijuana?

<u>Why indeed?</u>

CHAPTER 10
DO YOU *REALLY* KNOW "MARIJUANA"

Michael Moore, Filmmaker & Author:
"Yes I support decriminalizing marijuana. Our drug laws are hypocritical...and often racist. These laws have locked up an obscene number of people and this must end. And marijuana laws are the dumbest."

Recently I had a discussion with a clerk at a local marijuana dispensary. His lack of understanding and general knowledge of the different terminology used to correctly identify the Wonder Weed's various iterations surprised me. All he seemed to know about were printed facts on twenty or so strains he was selling, not in itself a bad thing.

On the assumption that a dispensary employee was relatively clueless about marijuana specifics, I presume that the general public is even more so. So I decided to write a short primer below in the hope my readers might find it interesting. Botanically:

- The entire hemp <u>FAMILY</u> is "cannabaceae".
- The cannabis <u>GENUS</u> is "hemp".
- All marijuana <u>SPECIES</u> are "cannabis sativa".

What is confusing is that **ALL** *four* primary marijuana plants are the <u>species</u> "cannabis sativa"! Also, *all* four marijuana plants are the *genus* hemp.

The hemp prohibition logic? Since hemp is marijuana it's the same "dangerous" plant as *any* and *all* marijuana. It isn't.

Charles Darwin made the point that the concept of "species" is just a human labeling system that gets in the way of seeing biological evolution as a gradual process of biodiversity. "If we do not forget this we can begin to make progress."

The cannabis plant evolved fifty million years ago, the last part of the age of the dinosaurs. Human-like creatures began to evolve less than *two* million years ago.

Each individual cannabis plant is either a male or a female. Without a mate the female flower will remain "unfinished", that is, without seed (called "sinsimilla", Spanish for : without=sin, similla=seed).

Male and female plants can be separated by a hundred miles or more and still reproduce! Male pollen is delivered to the sticky thick resin, full of cannabinoids , that exudes from near the female plant's sex organs. The male plant can produce over a BILLION grains of pollen in a season. They are tiny and light and can travel hundreds of miles on the wind. In its natural environment marijuana completes its entire life cycle in a single season. It is an "annual", like a petunia!

Marijuana is known to contain over four-hundred different compounds, including 87 cannabinoids *other than* the primary psychoactive component THC! The plant has always been cultivated for one of <u>three</u> useful products:

1. The nutritious seeds. The seeds are rich in oils and protein and have been used for thousands of years as human food, animal feed, fuel and skin care products.

2. The fibrous stalks. These have also been used for many centuries to make a very tough cloth, rope, and paper.

3. The resinous flowers. These have been used recreationally and medicinally for *thousands* of years. Cannabis resin contains chemical compounds known

as "cannabinoids", of which THC is the major psychoactive component. The desired product is large, dense buds of un-pollinated female sinsemilla flowers.

There is considerable debate among botanists and taxonomists over the exact classification of various marijuana plants. The following is an accurate simplification of the cannabis sativa sub-species spectrum.

There are four "pure" (read:"un-hybridized") varieties of cannabis sativa:

- **Indica - marijuana** variety of cannabis sativa. Its derivative products are used primarily for reduction of chronic pain. It is also used by insomniacs to induce sleep. Known as "nighttime weed", Indicas essentially relax nerves and create a sense of serenity. It is often said that "Indicas get you stoned".

- **Sativa- marijuana** variety of cannabis sativa. Used primarily to create an uplifting "high", this "daytime weed" stimulates appetite. It is used by cancer patients to reduce the nausea associated with chemotherapy.

- **Sativa- hemp** variety of cannabis sativa. **Note that all hemp is cannabis sativa, but all cannabis sativa is not hemp!** This creates a lot of confusion. Hemp is the industrial – use plant. (See Chapter 12). It grows wild throughout the mid-western United States where it is known as "ditch weed".

- **Ruderalis- marijuana variety of cannabis sativa.** This Asian variety has certain desirable growing traits, among which is cold-hardiness. It is almost useless for medical and recreational use because it is very low in the psychoactive and medicinal chemicals. It is often hybridized with Indica-marijuana and Sativa-marijuana plants because of the favorable growth characteristics.

As pointed out above, what has led over the years to the misunderstandings about hemp if the fact that **ALL HEMP IS CANNABIS SATIVA, BUT NOT ALL CANNABIS SATIVA IS HEMP!** Referring to common industrial hemp rope as "dope rope" hasn't exactly helped hemp's image either.

Equally confusing is that Indica-marijuana, Sativa-marijuana, Ruderalis-marijuana and Sativa-hemp are ALL part of the genus "**HEMP**"! No wonder industrial hemp has been illegal for so long! *Any* marijuana can correctly be called "hemp".

What totally complicates the entire marijuana picture is that *thousands* of hybrid strains of Indica-marijuana and Sativa-marijuana with some Ruderalis-marijuana often included exist today. These can have an infinite range of THC and CBD percentages, and on top of that an equally large range of terpene (see below) percentages and other chemicals.

You can find anything from 50/50 THC/CBD to 60/40, 70/30, 80/20, 90/10, 10/90, 20/80, 30/70, 40/60…and anything in between. Terpenes can be from almost zero to as much as 15% or so. Bioflavonoids are also present in smaller amounts, as are hundreds of other trace chemicals.

It is this *huge* range of sub-species, sub-sub-species (sub-sub….ad infinitum) that makes any effort by the federal government to create a "standard legal strain" for scientific testing for the effects on various maladies absolutely absurd.

This is why *only* a compilation of anecdotal testimonies from actual users as to the strains that have been effective for their particular needs is a practical, albeit

"un-scientific", way to correlate various strains as to their effectiveness for different maladies.

To cloud the picture further, the exact same strain can have very different medical effects on two users with the precisely same malady. Individual physiologies differ.

Let's take a look at the terpenes. They are the important compounds that give different marijuana strains their individually distinctive odors. They do the same for roses and all other flowers. Terpenes have been used for centuries in aromatherapy. They are best inhaled with a vaporizer.

Present in all marijuana (although the sativa-hemp variety of cannabis sativa has very few terpenes) they are a *major* contributor to the therapeutic effects found by patients to be of value for a long list of ailments. They act *synergistically* with the other cannabinoid chemicals present, enhancing some, depressing others.

There has not been as much published research on terpenes as on THC and CBD. I do know personally of a young PhD candidate in Australia who is dedicating herself to terpene research. Much work needs to be done in this area in the future. Terpene research is beyond a doubt at least as important as research into the medical effects of various ratios of THC and CBD.

There are sixteen primary terpenes, found in different marijuana strains in varying quantities. Terpenes can represent fifteen percent or so of the major marijuana constituents, which is quite significant.

The fourteen most common marijuana terpenes, in order of general amount found are (with some of the possible reported medicinal applications):

- beta-Myrcene: Earthy aroma. Pain killer, anti-inflammatory and antibiotic. This is most prevalent terpene found in most marijuana, but is not found in hemp. It apparently enters the blood stream, passes through the blood-brain barrier, and allows the psychoactive THC to act faster.

- Linalool : Floral aroma, spicy overtones. Anxiety relief; acne. It is the most powerful sedative of all the terpenes, and the second in importance.

- alpha-Terpineol: Lilac/citrus aroma. Partly responsible for "body highs". It acts synergistically with Linalool. It is an anti-depressant that reduces anxiety, and should have specific applications in PTSD patients.

- delta-Limonene: Orange aroma. Mood enhancer. Anti-bacterial, anti-fungal and anti-cancer activities are reported.

- alpha-Terpineol: Lilac/citrus aroma. It is reported to have antibiotic, antioxidant, and antimalarial properties.

- alpha-Humulene: Aroma of hops. Said to reduce inflammation.

- Caryophyllene oxide: Spicy aroma. Also said to repair nervous system damage.

- beta-Caryophyllene: Strong spicy aroma. Gastro-protective. Has anti-inflammatory properties.

- alpha-Pinene: Pine scent. Reported to act as a

bronchodilator.

- Terpinolene: Smoky wood aroma. Said to be anti-bacterial.

- Cineole: Eucalyptus odor. Pain relief, increases circulation.

- Puelgone: Said to have sedative effects.

- Eucalyptol: Eucalyptus odor. A stimulant with anti-inflammatory properties.

- p-Cymene: Said to be an antibiotic.

Note that there is a *huge* difference between consuming raw marijuana, and heating it before consumption. The components in raw marijuana are converted ONLY through heating into the compounds THC and CBD that we commonly attribute to marijuana's potency and effectiveness.

While specific benefits and effects are attributed to raw un-heated marijuana, a different, and somewhat longer list of attributes are found with the heated product. The raw plants contain THCA, or tetrahydrocannabinollic acid, and CBDA, cannabanollic acid, which convert to THC and CBD upon heating.

We also find many other cannabinoids in marijuana, the most common being:

- Cannabigerol (CBG): This is a non-psychoactive cannabinoid with many sub-types. It has been found to be a more potent pain killer than THC, is anti-microbial, and shown effective against psoriasis and depression. Some strains contain as high as 4% CBG. Behind THC and CBD it is the third most common cannabinoid found in various strains.

- Cannabichromine (CBC): It is more abundant in immature plants, and has many sub-types. It is not as highly studied as other cannabinoids, but significant amounts appear in some potent varieties.

- Cannabitriol (CBT): Has been noted as present in male flowers, and in some Asian marijuanas. and some hashish.

- Cannabielsoin (CBE): Is a derivative of CBD. I could find no specific studies.

- Cannabinol (CBN): This is created by degradation of THCA after harvest. It can be created if marijuana is pressed into blocks (think Mexico) where the resin glands are crushed allowing oxidation. It is not a desirable component because it exaggerates THC's disorienting qualities.

Potency of any given marijuana strain is a direct factor of genetics. Different strains of marijuana are characterized by:

- Height
- Width
- Branching traits
- Leaf size
- Leaf shape
- Time to reach flowering
- Potency
- Taste

- Type of high
- Aroma
- Medicinal benefits

Mature Sativa-marijuana plants are actually *trees* that commonly grow up to 12 feet tall, and *can* achieve 20 feet! They have the conical shape of Christmas trees. In contrast Indicas are more dense and bush-like. They mature more quickly than Sativas and are rarely over 6 feet high.

While easy to see the difference between mature plants it is very hard to tell the difference when looking at buds in a dispensary jar.

Pure Indica buds are usually thick and dense and dark green to purple, and are roundish in shape. Pure Sativa buds are generally long and thin, and can range in color from orange, red and purple, or even light green. Hybrid strains can have the characteristics of each and are hard to identify by sight.

Buyers of marijuana should be aware that it doesn't "keep" very well. It changes as it ages, with considerations for *how* it is stored. Temperature, humidity, light conditions, and how well oxygen is sealed out are factors. That is not to say that "aged" marijuana does not have useful properties. It is just that they will differ somewhat from fresh product whether either one is consumed raw or heated.

There is one point I would like to make in an effort to refute the oft-stated fallacy (read: media lie) that "marijuana today is much stronger than it was in the '70s". Typical headline: "It's Not Your Grandpa's Pot!" This is only *partly* true, and *barely* so. For the most part present-day highly available street marijuana is much weaker than grandpa's.

As an example, two pure basic "original" '70s strains, known as "land races", were Panama Red and Columbian Gold. Their psychoactive cannabinoid content, the percentage of THC, was _higher_ than almost all of the marijuana strains sold today even in legal dispensaries.

Compared to common Mexican street-marijuana available everywhere in the United States, these '70s strains were MUCH more powerful. At the time THEY were the common street marijuana, and they were quite potent!

It **is** true, however, that a few hybrids have been created today that have THC content as high as 30% or more. They are available at some dispensaries, but I am told they are NOT top sellers. They are certainly not a sufficient reason for the effort in the media to make marijuana seem like it is a far greater, stronger "threat" than it ever was in the past. It isn't.

With thousands of strains, and hundreds of cannabinoids and terpenes and their various oxidation products, and various ways to use the products, it is abundantly clear that true scientific research cannot possibly be applied to every possible iteration of all these many variables.

It would take a hundred years of massive research to even scratch the surface of the theoretically possible scientific studies. Clearly there is no _immediate_ need for more studies. These can wait.

In the interest of all of our suffering and dying citizens **we need decriminalization and legalization NOW!**

CHAPTER 11
MARIJUANA vs BIG TOBACCO
AND BIG ALCOHOL

Morgan Freeman, Actor, Academy Award Winner,
Marijuana Activist:
"It's just the stupidest law possible. You're just making criminals out of people who aren't engaged in criminal activity. And we're spending zillions of dollars trying to fight a war we can't win! We could make zillions, just legalize it and tax it like we do liquor. It's stupid."

The huge pharmaceutical companies clearly stand to be the big losers once medical marijuana becomes mainstream. They have spent billions of dollars spreading anti-marijuana propaganda for decades. Politicians, physicians and the media have turned their backs to the truth at the beck and call of Big Pharma.

What about the OTHER two big *killers* (besides prescription opioids) tobacco and alcohol? We tried alcohol prohibition for over a decade and all it got us was marijuana prohibition. We've had a War On Drugs since Nixon declared it and we have more and deadlier street drugs available today than ever before. The United States is not real good at protecting its citizens from themselves,

It is often said that the only difference between smoking cigarettes and smoking marijuana is that cigarettes make Uncle Sam rich (taxes) and marijuana costs Uncle Sam money (enforcement/incarceration expenses.) This is not exactly the *only* difference. There is a far more important difference. **Tobacco kills. Marijuana does not.**

The American Cancer society estimates that a **half million**

Americans die each year from smoking-related cancers. Countless studies have shown that there is NO equivalent situation with marijuana. None. Some Israeli and other studies even suggest marijuana as a <u>cancer preventative</u>! Studies sponsored by the tobacco industry lobby obviously show the exact opposite result. What a surprise!

Big money talks, loud. It is not only Big Pharma's billions of lobbying cash and perks that have dominated for decades. How exactly do you think Big Tobacco and Big Alcohol have managed to remain off the federal drug Schedules *entirely*? Do you believe that either of these huge industries care at all about government-mandated "warning labels"? These warnings mean very little to the all-mighty bottom line.

So why not add alcohol and tobacco to the drug Schedules? Past history. The 18th Amendment to the United States Constitution classified alcohol as a disease causative. Prohibition was law. And no one gave a damn!

Alcohol was available everywhere, to anyone, mostly provided by organized crime, some by home-brewing. There was no alcohol tax revenue coming in. After fourteen long years of prohibition, and the storied efforts of Eliot Ness and his "Untouchables", the 18th Amendment had to be repealed. Ness was now "Unemployable"! Prohibition simply didn't work, just as today's War On Drugs doesn't work.

The United States government every year collects over a staggering $6,000,000,000 (that's six BILLION) tax dollars related to alcoholic beverages! Surely there is very little sentiment for losing even a part of *this* revenue stream.

Today alcohol and tobacco combined are responsible for a **quarter-TRILLION dollars in annual sales!** Aside from raising billions in taxes, it creates hundreds of thousands of jobs. Would it be in America's best interest to reschedule **these** as Schedule I? It's all in the viewpoint.

The World Health Organization states that worldwide every year alcohol consumption directly kills about 150,000 people, and is responsible for over **three million** alcohol-related fatalities. They further state that there are over seventeen million alcohol addicts in the United States alone at present. These are startling numbers!

One of the common arguments for not legalizing marijuana goes like this: "OK, we accept that smoking tobacco products kills many thousands of people by cancer each year. Very sad. We accept that alcohol kills, directly and indirectly. But *three* wrongs do not make a right. Why add yet another killer to the ones that already exist?"

Why? Because there is absolutely <u>no valid comparison</u> between tobacco smokers, alcohol users, and marijuana users, that would indicate against legalization. Let me explain.

For starters, there is no nicotine in marijuana. None. So this very harmful addictive chemical is immediately removed from the equation. Score one for legalization.

Here is the most important distinction between tobacco and marijuana. It relates to the **quantity** of smoke that is normally inhaled. **The contrast is stunning.** It is a fact that it takes **very little** marijuana smoke to achieve *any* desired effect, medicinal or pleasurable.   Many studies have also proven beyond a doubt that marijuana smoking is NOT addictive. On the other hand, the smoke inhaled by the average tobacco nicotine-addicted smoker is FAR greater in quantity. *Tobacco smoking **is** addictive.*

A cigarette smoker can easily inhale the smoke from an ounce or more (generally a *lot* more) of tobacco **every single day.** **It is rare for a marijuana smoker to consume an ounce in an entire MONTH!**

A one-pack-a-day smoker (double it for the two-packer) consumes 20 cigarettes a pack. On average each cigarette is good for 10 lungsful of smoke. That's 200 (or 400) lungsful of smoke every single day. The point is, puff for puff marijuana smoke may (or may not) be just as harmful as tobacco smoke. It is simply critical to note that the NUMBER of puffs of marijuana smoke is almost *insignificant* in comparison.

Does Big Pharma have a dog in the tobacco and alcohol fight? Of course they do. A large dog! They sell billions of dollars of medications related to alcohol consumption and addiction. These include the benzodiazepine compounds (such as diazepam), and other drugs such as disulfram, haltrexone and acamprostate.

How about tobacco? We have nicotine patches. We have nicotine pills. We have similar anti-addiction drugs as for alcohol. The last thing in the world that Big Pharma would ever want to see is a serious reduction in alcohol and tobacco addiction. Surely there is zero sentiment to lose the massive profits from supplying these anti-addiction wonder drugs.

Marijuana legalization is beyond a doubt a major threat to the bottom-line profitability of Big Pharma. On the valid assumption that many who now turn to alcohol will decide instead to use marijuana, Big Alcohol's bottom line could suffer as well. What about Big Tobacco?

Tobacco companies grow zillions of acres of tobacco plants. Big Tobacco's executives are salivating over the possible conversion of these crops to marijuana! They have *already* copyrighted many names for entire product lines of marijuana-based cigarettes. They can hardly wait!

On a per-acre basis cultivation of marijuana could prove to be more profitable than tobacco. So Big Tobacco has far less to fear from marijuana legalization than do either Big Pharma or Big Alcohol.

Quite recently the federal government decided to "crack down" on ALL forms of tobacco and tobacco substitutes. They have decided to mandate serious warnings similar to those on cigarette packages. This will now include pipe tobacco, cigars, chewing tobacco and, incredibly, tobacco-substitute vape pens!

Does the tobacco industry really care about this "smoke screen" (bad pun intended)? Why should they? Severe ad restrictions and warning labels have been around for decades, and they still make billions in profits.

Could this "increased pressure" on Big Tobacco be a prelude to an even stronger crackdown on marijuana? Does it matter? Does anyone who is addicted to nicotine actually pay any attention at all to package warnings?

Of course not.

CHAPTER 12
WHAT ABOUT HEMP?

<u>Thomas Jefferson,</u> United States President:
"Hemp is of first necessity to the wealth and protection of the country. The greatest service that can be rendered to any country is to add a useful plant to its culture."

<u>Pamela Anderson</u>, Actress and Model:
"I think we should legalize marijuana, tax and monitor, farm hemp, etc. This would make our borders less corrupt and then I think eventually this will be a more secure option and save children in the long run. It would create jobs and be good for the environment."

GOD said: "See, I give you every seed bearing plant that is upon all the earth....they shall be yours for food". Genesis 1:29

IS ANYONE OUT THERE LISTENING?

The industrial hemp plant is the sativa-hemp variety of cannabis sativa. "Hemp" is also the botanical genus of ALL cannabis plants. This includes the three marijuana varieties, Indica-marijuana, Sativa-marijuana, and Ruderalis-marijuana.

In the 1980s an author named Jack Herer, a major advocate for legalization, had a profound influence in differentiating industrial hemp from the other more psychoactive forms of marijuana. His book, *The Emperor Wears No Clothes,* was a very detailed history of 3,000 years of using hemp in dozens of useful ways. Apparently no one in political power can read.

There is no other natural soft fiber known on earth that exhibits the durability and strength of hemp fiber. It has been used in the sail cloth and rigging of sailing ships since sailing ships were invented! For almost two hundred years from the 1630s to the 1800s hemp was actually accepted in America as legal tender. Even taxes could be paid with it!

This incentive was offered to inspire farmers to plant hemp instead of tobacco. George Washington and Thomas Jefferson owned hemp farms. There was even a time when a farmer could be jailed for NOT cultivating hemp!

After the United States Congress in 1937 passed the federal prohibition of "mari*hu*ana" (gotta keep it Mexican) it put all of the domestic hemp producers out of business along with all of the manufacturers of legal cannabis medicines. Apparently the feds never got the news that sativa-hemp was NOT psychoactive marijuana. After all, it WAS Sativa.

During WWII the United States government actually provided farmers with 200 tons of hemp seed! This allowed farmers to produce 42,000 tons of hemp fiber during the war. The Department of Agriculture oversaw the production of 300,000 acres of hemp plants throughout Iowa, Minnesota, Illinois, Wisconsin, Kentucky and Indiana.

The Japanese controlled most of the South Pacific hemp production. America desperately needed hemp for rope rigging and canvas cloth. Even parachutes were made of hemp canvas. Once the war ended, hemp was again illegal. Brilliant move.

Here are some of the common industrial uses for hemp:

- Fuel. Hemp acts the same as corn or waste paper

when it comes to biomass. It can be converted to alcohol to power vehicles.

- Concrete. Known as "hempcrete", mixed into concrete it creates a product that weighs half as much, and is more durable.

- Food. Hemp seeds are a great source of protein and essential amino acids.

- Fabrics. Hemp cloth has been used for decades to make clothing. It was used in antiquity to make sails. The "covered wagons" that settled the west were covered in hemp cloth. It was used in WWII to make parachutes. The earliest known fabrics are hemp cloth from China made 10,000 years ago! "Canvas" derives from the same root as "cannabis".

- Oil. Hemp oil is used in many cosmetic products. It makes a tasty salad dressing. It can have proven healing properties because of the non-psychoactive cannabidiol (CBD) present.

  Do not be misled when you read the label on a bottle of hemp oil. The federal government has cracked down on any written label suggestion that the oil might actually *have* some therapeutic value. Idiots.

- Rope. "Dope rope" has been used since the dawn of civilization. It was used to tie together early rafts. It was used for centuries as boat rigging. (Connecting hemp with "dope", a generic name for illegal drugs, does not exactly help hemp's overall legalization efforts!)

- Paper. The Declaration of Independence was written on hemp paper. Its value for paper was partially to blame for the entire criminalization of marijuana in the 1930's. William Randolph Hearst had huge interests in forestry and news-printing paper, and saw hemp as a major threat. This is not unlike Big Pharma seeing a similar financial threat from marijuana today.

Incredibly, until recently it was illegal to grow hemp anywhere in the United States. Completely ignoring *analyses* proving that hemp contains almost no psychoactive components, the mere fact that it is *related* botanically to marijuana was enough for Uncle Sam to ban farmers from growing it nationwide for decades. Truly brain dead.

What is even stupider is that all products containing hemp and hemp oil were always perfectly legal to *sell* in the USA! The hemp used just has to be ***grown* somewhere else!** Is there any *end* to our government's stupidity? Apparently not.

Hemp production has the potential to be a **multi-billion dollar industry** that can bring in hundreds of millions in tax revenue. It can create hundreds of thousands of new jobs. How blind can our government officials be? Very.

Obviously, as with Big Pharma and marijuana legalization, powerful lobby groups in the timber and paper industry have somehow (guess how?) managed to sway political opinion away from hemp growing legalization since the end of WWII. Add this as being yet another **national disgrace**.

About twelve years ago the Drug Enforcement Agency (DEA) began formulating guidelines for domestic hemp growth. In 2014 a Farm Bill *finally* allowed state agricultural departments to set up experimental hemp farms using DEA-certified seeds Hemp plants produce some cannabidiol (CBD), the non-psychoactive cannabinoid. CBD is a potent medicine for many conditions, and may eventually prove to be by far the most important research medicine.

Hemp plants produce less than 1% of the psychoactive component THC. One strike against a hemp crop is that physically it is almost indistinguishable from a crop of THC-laden marijuana plants. This leaves open the possibility of some illegal crops containing a mix of hemp cannabis plants and marijuana cannabis plants to be grown together and difficult to detect.

The general public is unaware that there is the hemp source of CBD in addition to CBD extracted from other marijuana plants. It is entirely legal to buy CBD laden hemp oil online and have it shipped anywhere in the United States. In fact pure hemp oil is readily available at most health food stores.

The irony is that marijuana-based CBD is illegal federally, while the hemp- based oil containing CBD is NOT a specifically Scheduled product and thereby legal. Only when CBD oil is derived from federally illegal marijuana plants does it fall under the inane Schedule I classification! Simply crazy.

This is not to say that the FDA, exercising its "protect the public at all costs" mandate, hasn't taken note of the hemp oil being sold legally in America. They have recently cracked down on specific health claims being put on labels, quite honestly, by some manufacturers.

I hope someday to see a good lab analysis of the CBD present in the commercial hemp oil that costs me $15.00 for a 16 ounce bottle at my local health food store. I'd like to see a side-by-side comparison with the $35.00 per 2 ounce tincture bottle that my medical marijuana dispensary sells me!

GW Pharmaceuticals in England produces the CBD/THC product Sativex mentioned earlier. They are seeking exclusive patent rights in the United States. It would seem to be difficult for them to prove that a natural herb in use for thousands of years that belongs to all humanity could be controlled by them exclusively. Should they prevail the CBD component from the hemp industry could have a very short life in America. *Why* might they succeed? Any guesses?

Anyone living anywhere in the United States, who believes that commercial hemp oil could be of some health benefit, should not hesitate to buy and use it. You don't need a "medical marijuana card". At least not yet.

If you *have* a card and live in a state where you can drop by your friendly local legal cannabis dispensary you can always buy the expensive seed-to-sale tracked CBD product there. You can be certain you will be getting a top quality hemp oil. It is FAR less expensive to visit a health food store or buy an equivalent product on line. My only caution is that you buy a major brand from one of the large public companies that cold-press the oil themselves.

It is very encouraging that some hemp is being grown now in the United States. The potential for this crop from all of its products listed above is massive in terms of tax revenues and jobs. It could well turn out that hemp becomes the primary cannabis crop, perhaps THE primary crop overall, in the United States in future years.

CHAPTER 13
ARGUMENTS AGAINST LEGALIZATION

Newt Gingrich, **Former Speaker of the U.S. House of Representatives and possible VP candidate:**
"No, you shouldn't be arrested for recreational drug use."

John Anderson, **Former Correctional Officer & Criminology Professor at Malaspina University- College:**
"It is a tragic irony that more people have died or been injured from the enforcement of marijuana laws than any harms generated from the herb itself. The negative costs to society are the result of the legal status of marijuana, not its pharmacological properties."

Any book about marijuana legalization must give space to the many arguments *against* legalization. It is a fact that virtually every argument against legalization has been based on ignorance of the truth due to decades of lies and government deceit. Regardless, I would be remiss were I not to give voice to the legion of dissenters. Here goes.

Fortunately, virtually every one of these anti-marijuana-arguments has been disproven through genuine scientific studies. Unfortunately one has to do considerable research to locate and verify these studies. Big Pharma has gone out of its way to spread enough cash and other perks around to insure that neither politicians nor doctors nor the media will ever be fully aware of the truth.

Remember the saying by Mark Twain: "It is easy to fool the people, but extremely hard to un-fool them." The American people have been fooled for decades. Here, in no particular order, is a litany of beliefs that are held by far too many "fooled" Americans, as well as legions of "fooled" doctors:

- Marijuana kills brain cells and makes you stupid;
- Marijuana will destroy your lungs;
- Marijuana smoking will makes you look terrible;
- Marijuana smokers experience dry mouth, bloodshot eyes, and swollen eyelids;
- Smoking marijuana while pregnant is very harmful. (No one will argue this point. But so are tobacco and alcohol, probably more so. Easy solution: Don't drink, smoke tobacco, or use marijuana if you are pregnant);
- You will cough uncontrollably.

Statistics show that far fewer than half of all marijuana users actually *smoke joints*. Most vape, use tinctures, or ingest edibles, and are thereby cough-free. Aside from smoking, the anti-marijuana crowd insists that:

- You will gain weight on marijuana;
- Marijuana causes dangerous hallucinations;
- Marijuana weakens the immune system;
- Use marijuana and end up in jail;
- Grow marijuana and end up in jail;
- Marijuana inhibits kids brain growth;
- Marijuana lowers IQ;
- Driving under the influence of marijuana will cause a huge spike in traffic accidents and deaths;
- Marijuana is a gateway drug to other more deadly drugs;
- You can die from using too much marijuana;
- Why add a third evil…alcohol and tobacco are enough;
- You will surely end up in the Emergency Ward;
- Marijuana will ruin your heart;
- Marijuana will ruin your kidneys and liver;
- Marijuana is addictive, just as cocaine and heroin;

- There is absolutely no need to legalize marijuana because a synthetic form, dronabinol, sold as Marinol, can be prescribed by doctors as a capsule;
- If marijuana is readily available and promoted as "medicine" kids will be more likely to try it because "medicine is good for you";
- Marijuana edibles are just too tempting for kids;
- Eating marijuana will surely kill your dog or cat;
- There are deadly pesticides and mold in marijuana;
- Kids will get hooked on marijuana as a "gateway drug";
- Second hand marijuana smoke is just as bad as actually smoking marijuana;
- Marijuana is not now and never will be covered by medical insurance;
- Marijuana will cause widespread bankruptcies;
- There is a huge social stigma to using marijuana;
- Marijuana will make you and your house stink;
- You can lose your job for using marijuana;
- When you buy marijuana from a street dealer you have no idea what you are getting;
- Marijuana today is *much* stronger and deadlier than it was years ago.

This is just a partial list! I have actually read each of these in the media from time to time. I'm certain any marijuana hater can think up others. If you can think of any others please email me and I will be sure to include them in my next edition! Please send to: burta193811@yahoo.com.

There *are* actual possible downsides to marijuana use. One is the real danger of using marijuana in conjunction with other prescription, over the counter, and illegal street drugs, and experiencing a bad reaction. For example when combined with:

- Theophylline: Reduced theophylline in the body;
- Disulfiram & Fluoxetine: Mild manic episodes;
- Cocaine: Increased heart rate and blood pressure;
- Amphetamines: Increased heart rate and blood pressure;
- Antihistamines: Increased heart rate and/or drowsiness;
- Tricyclic antidepressants: Increased heart rate, blood pressure and drowsiness;
- Barbituates and depressant sedatives: Causes too much sleepiness;
- Alcohol and other sedatives: Increased drowsiness. (Because the THC molecule is soluble in alcohol use of marijuana in conjunction with drinking *any* alcoholic beverage, including beer, will *greatly* magnify the effect of marijuana);
- Prozac: Irritability, nervousness, excitability.

To research drug-drug interactions check out the website: http://www.rxlist.com. There have actually been very few good studies of the interaction of marijuana consumed in conjunction with a wide range of prescription and illegal drugs.

For all intents and purposes it is a very bad idea to take *any* medications when using marijuana. It is also highly recommended that anyone with heart disease, pulmonary disease, schizophrenia or is pregnant should consult their physician before trying any form of marijuana.

Thanks to the information published in a brochure from the University of Arizona, occasional marijuana side effects could include:

- Shortness of breath;
- Dizziness when rising;
- Change of heart rate, rarely arrhythmia;
- Tremors;
- Pancreatitis (rare);
- Difficult urination;
- Vision changes;
- Anxiety;
- Unsteadiness walking;
- Slurred speech;
- Disorientation;
- Depression;
- Paranoia;
- Lack of motivation;
- Panic attacks;
- Headache;
- Mood swings;
- Hallucinations;
- Memory problems;
- Fainting.

Of course the vast majority of these, even if they do occur, which is rare, usually pass in a few hours.

Not to be outdone, the federal Drug Enforcement Agency (DEA) has its own truly idiotic list of ten damning marijuana-related problems:

1. Crime, violence and marijuana use go hand in hand.

2. Significant progress has been made in the war on drugs --- let's not stop now.

3. Legalization of marijuana will lead to increased use and increased addiction.

4. Any tax revenues will evaporate due to increased social costs.

5. No compelling medical reasons to prescribe marijuana.

6. Legalization and decriminalization in other countries a dismal failure.

7. Drug control spending is only a tiny part of the US budget.

8. Drug prohibition is working.

9. Drug legalization would have an adverse effect on low income communities.

10. Home insurance may well be impacted, especially if you have an indoor or outdoor grow facility.

While we are at it, let's hear from the Food and Drug Administration (FDA). The FDA requires five criteria to be fulfilled for any drug to be scheduled higher than marijuana's Schedule I:

1. The drug's chemistry must be known and reproducible. This includes purity, dosage, and shelf life.

2. There must be adequate safety studies.

3. There must be adequate and well-controlled studies providing efficacy.

4. The drug must be accepted by well-qualified experts.

5. Scientific evidence must be widely available.

The ten DEA arguments and five FDA arguments have been so thoroughly disproven through decades of scientific study as to not being worthy of further comment in this Chapter. Most are covered elsewhere in this book.

I really hope this Chapter makes the anti-marijuana crowd happy! Maybe I even suggested to some a bit of new ammunition! I also hope they read and try to understand the information in the next Chapter, which refutes most of the negatives with actual scientific studies. (Also see Chapter 15)

What we are dealing here is simply a question of: **"Do the positives outweigh any *possible* negatives?"**

What to me makes the argument for legalization irrefutable is that it is very difficult to quantify human suffering. It is easier to ignore it.

America has ignored it for far too long.

CHAPTER 14
ARGUMENTS FOR LEGALIZATION

<u>John H. Richardson</u>, Writer-at-Large for Esquire, &
Author:
"The drug war isn't just a failure. It's a spectacular failure.
An arrest will hurt your chances of getting a job or a
college loan or even a car loan, which will help push you
into a more marginalized existence, if not a life of full-time
criminality. In Mexico, in the last five years, police and
drug cartels have killed more than 55,000 people. Now the
Department of Justice says that drug cartels are running
drug-distribution networks in over 1,000 U.S. cities and
growing marijuana in national forests. With legal
marijuana, America will see an explosion of farms, stores,
and manufacturing facilities for everything from potency-
testing kits to specialized agricultural equipment."

<u>Melissa Etheridge</u>, Singer, Grammy Winner, Activist:
"It's wrong to arrest adults for using marijuana, and it's
even more wrong to allow gangs and cartels to profit
from selling marijuana. Instead, we should allow adults to
possess limited amounts of marijuana and we should
regulate marijuana sales in order to generate tax
revenues for public school construction and other
community needs. To me, regulating marijuana is simply
the right thing to do."

After reading the preceding Chapter one could easily
conclude that marijuana is in fact the "Devil's Weed". There
are so many theoretical and hypothetical arguments against it
that continued prohibition seems to be a no-brainer. **That is,
until you know the truth.**

The reality is that if you take ANY *legal* drug and create the same sorts of lists of negatives you will end up with lists that are *at least* as bad. In fact, there is one single critical word **absent** from the list of marijuana's negatives: **"DEATH". You can say what you want about marijuana, but you cannot correctly say that anyone in human history has ever died from an overdose. That is not true of ANY other drug.**

Aside from its safety, marijuana has been proven for thousands of years to have an incredible range of medicinal properties. In Chapters 15 and 17 I try to show the validity of this statement. If my readers choose they can do further study by actually accessing the hundreds of scientific papers referenced in books I have listed.

The evidence in favor of legalization, both anecdotal and scientifically verified, is overwhelming. Marijuana can in fact alleviate pain and suffering, and replace a wide range of truly addictive and deadly products. It is this quality alone that makes the arguments for legalization of marijuana far more persuasive than all of the arguments for prohibition combined!

There are many other reasons that can be added to the "it cannot kill" and "it definitely is a proven medicine" arguments:

- Statistics show that far fewer than half of all marijuana users actually *smoke joints*. Most vape, use tinctures, or ingest edibles. This fact eliminates ALL of the arguments that relate to *smoking* marijuana for at least half of the present and future users;

- Throughout history marijuana has brought people together. Virtually the entire jazz community in the '30s smoked marijuana. Almost all of the hundreds of thousands of "Hippies" in the '60s used marijuana.

Many entertainers today are drawn together through common use of this harmless healing wonder herb.

- Many of the arguments against marijuana are rooted in racism. The word "marihuana" came into popular use because it sounded "Mexican", and Mexicans were vilified and despised. It is more commonly spelled "marijuana" today. Americans in the '30s were "taught" to hate blacks and Mexicans by Anslinger and Hearst. They learned well.

- Legalize marijuana and you remove one more tool used against minorities. Legalizing marijuana could help unite the races rather than alienate them from each other.

It is sad but true that a criminal record virtually never goes away. It is in the public record forever. In this computer age it is very simple for anyone to learn about an individual's past indiscretions. Websites such as instantcheckmate.com legally make such information readily available.

It is also sad but true that many, if not most, employers will hesitate to hire anyone with a criminal record or any sort. Possession and/or sale of marijuana is one such "crime". Decriminalization of marijuana would open countless doors of employment opportunity to many inner-city youths who presently are virtually unemployable because of their arrests for using or selling a harmless herbal medicine.

- Prison populations would drop dramatically. In the latest year with solid statistics, of 872,772 people were incarcerated for marijuana convictions. They were disproportionately black. 775,137 were for *simple possession*. Often this is as little as an ounce or less.

Not only would it end the gross injustice of these incarcerations, but hundreds of prisons could be closed resulting in billions of dollars saved. Of course the huge private prison industry (Big Prison) is yet another lobby group strongly against decriminalization. It could well put many of them out of business.

- Legalization would eliminate entire categories of victimless crimes. The most violent crimes linked to marijuana profit motives would decrease. The police could then focus limited resources on real felonies.

- Our greatly overburdened courts will be relieved of the problem of hundreds of thousands of minor marijuana offenses to be ajudicated.

- Good old Uncle Sam stands to get billions of dollars more in tax revenue than they get today. The use of taxes generated by legalization could be channeled into kids' anti-street-drug educational programs.

- The states, most of which are struggling with entitlement program spending and unfunded pensions, would earn millions in new tax revenue.

- Millions of _new_ jobs will be created. These jobs never existed before legalization. (See Chapter 32).

- Border violence, especially in Arizona, Texas and California, would significantly decrease. The demand for Mexican marijuana could be eliminated if legal marijuana is properly controlled and priced.

- Because marijuana is now sold illegally everywhere, it

is just as easy for kids to get ahold of it as it is for adults. Making it legal with the same restrictions as tobacco and alcohol will make access by youths far more difficult.

- If marijuana is legalized it will be a first step towards easing the absurd premise that declaring a "WAR" on everything will solve anything.

- Almost every marijuana users partakes in order to "escape" something. This reasoning is shared with alcohol consumption. But marijuana is not nearly as addictive or deadly as alcohol. It is not nearly as detrimental in terms of violence while under its influence. If made legal it stands to reason that people would drink less and get high more! Fewer drunks = fewer drunk drivers = fewer drunk-driving accidents.

- There are estimated to be a half-million deaths a year directly due to smoking cigarettes. Marijuana contains fewer known-harmful chemicals than tobacco, and can be wrapped in hemp paper to preclude inhaling burnt paper smoke.

  More important, marijuana smokers smoke FAR FEWER joints than the average cigarette smoker consumes cigarettes, possibly 95% fewer! No one smokes two packs of joints a day! Two joints, period, is more realistic.

Anti-legalization activists cite the dangers of marijuana as the top reason it should be kept illegal. But way back in 1972 the National Commission on Marihuana and Drug Use concluded that the dangers of smoking marijuana had been "grossly overstated".

In 1995 the respected British medical journal Lancet, based on scientific studies, reported: "<u>The smoking of marijuana, even long term, is not harmful to health</u>".

- It has been proven that fewer than ten percent of heavy, habitual marijuana users become truly addicted. This is lower than any deadly street drug, and lower than almost all prescription medicines such as opioids. It is FAR LESS addictive than alcohol or tobacco.

One of my closest friends has been a heavy marijuana smoker since 1970. As with all long term users he has built up a tolerance. I recently saw him smoke eight joints in a row and show absolutely no sign of loss of any faculty. Is he addicted? Every two years or so he goes cold turkey for a few months. Does he crave a joint AT ALL during that time? He swears he does not. Is he addicted? You tell me.

- Illegal Mexican marijuana is available *anywhere* in the United States. It *often* contains harmful adulterants, mold and bacteria. Legalize and regulate marijuana as we do tobacco and alcohol and at the very least you reduce the consumption of the potentially-harmful Mexican street-marijuana.

- Legalization in parts of the United States, and the very high quality of marijuana grown in Colorado and somehow ending up for use in Mexico, has actually slowed Mexican marijuana production! Many ex-marijuana farmers are changing crops, switching to a

Mexican government subsidized vegetable growing program. Unfortunately some have chosen to grow heroin poppies instead of tomatoes!

- Legalization, and universal availability of quality, controlled marijuana will greatly reduce the use of deadly Chinese designer street drugs by our youths. (See Chapter 23)

- The extensive use of harmful addictive opiates to relieve pain could be almost completely eliminated! This will save thousands of lives each year. It will at last allow our brave PTSD afflicted veterans the non-addictive relief they deserve. Prince might be alive.

- The unrestricted recreational use of marijuana will reduce the recreational use of harmful and addictive alcohol and tobacco.

- There are virtually NO adverse long-tern side effects from marijuana use except those traced to the use of contaminated Mexican product.

I mention "long term" because I have not seen a single anecdotal report of ANY such ill effects whatsoever. With thousands of years of marijuana experience, one could conclude that if there were any serious long-term problems they most surely would have been reported by now with the media hungry to damn marijuana, truth or not!

- Legal marijuana is expensive and not covered by insurance. Clearly, as regular market forces of supply and demand take hold prices will inevitably drop. This is seen already in many legalization states. The good news is that the first glimmer of insurance coverage hope has <u>already occurred</u>!

A tiny but critical step, one that might have far-reaching implications, occurred recently. Sun Life Insurance (Canada) was persuaded to pay the costs of medical marijuana for a student at Waterloo University, under their existing medical policy! This is not to say that BIG INSURANCE doesn't have their own reasons for lobbying heavily against legalization. Hope springs eternal!

- Marijuana has been proven in scientific study after study that it is NOT a so-called "gateway drug". It is often cited that kids will get hooked on marijuana and move on to far worse drugs.

Consider these questions: Do kids today ever smoke tobacco? Do kids today ever drink beer and alcohol? Do kids today ever sniff glue? Do kids today ever experiment with deadly designer street drugs? **Of course they do, on all counts.**

Kids always have and they always will. Can all these products kill? YES! Can marijuana kill? NO. Point made. The fact is that availability of quality, non-contaminated marijuana could greatly <u>REDUCE</u> the deadly use of street drugs by our vulnerable youth.

Some claim that smoking marijuana is harmful to the lungs. It is well documented that, although marijuana has been smoked extensively for decades, there is not a <u>single reported case</u> of emphysema or lung cancer attributed to marijuana. Dr. Lester Ginspoon of Harvard Medical School is quoted as saying: "I suspect that a day's breathing in any city with poor air quality poses more of a threat than inhaling a day's dose of marijuana."

There is one common lie about marijuana that has been spread for decades. It sticks in people's minds and seems to many to be a valid reason to continue marijuana prohibition. This is the erroneous contention that marijuana today is "far more potent", and thereby far more dangerous, than "grandpa's marijuana". This is a **total lie**.

The original eight classic strains imported by Marijuana Inc. in the '70s were: Acaculco Gold, Columbian Gold, Panama Red, Thai Stick, Durban Poison (South Africa), Lamb's Bread (Jamaica); Maui Wowee (HI), and Matanuska Thunderfuck (AK).

These all had far higher percentages of THC that most of the marijuana sold legally in dispensaries today, as well as illegal Mexican street crap. It *is* true that some marijuana medicinal strains, available only from dispensaries under carefully controlled conditions, have been highbredized to have a greater THC content. Dispensary owners tell me that these are *far* from being their better selling products.

New strains are **not** created in a mad rush to see how high a percentage of psychoactive THC can be offered. Strains are created to produce a wide range of *desirable* characteristics, not the least of which are aroma and physical appearance. Grandpa's marijuana was FAR more potent!

Let's depart from marijuana for a moment to reinforce a point. Most serious baseball fans know all about Tyrus "Ty" Cobb. Yes, he was undeniably great. His statistics and records that stand after almost a century prove it. But he is best known as a horrible person, a dedicated racist. A total reprobate.

Cobb cheated as a base runner. He was "known" to sharpen

his spikes with a file and deliberately try to injure opponents as he was sliding into any base. He was just an awful person by any measure.   There are even two published biographies that prove *conclusively* that he was one seriously nasty human being!

When one looks deeply into the facts, **_NONE_ OF THIS IS TRUE**! For starters, the biographies were pure fiction, in fact written by an individual with a personal axe to grind. He hated Cobb. They were simply total lies. The well-known "racial incident" where Cobb rushed into the stands and beat the crap out of two hecklers was true.....except the guys were WHITE, not black as widely reported. This fabrication is one of many believed to this day.

Confirmed interviews with teammates and competitors alike invariably described him as a perfect gentleman who NEVER tried to injure an opponent with a slide. Yet his legacy as a mean, dirty racist has persevered for decades.

Be it Tyrus Cobb - the Wonder Player, or *Marijuana – The Wonder Weed*, the media can plant an impression in the minds of Americans that is totally the opposite of reality, and **very hard to erase.**

What we have with marijuana legalization is a "risk vs reward" model. Most of the arguments against legalization can be mitigated with plain old common sense. Most of the others have been conclusively proven false through media-suppressed scientific studies.

As I suggest throughout this book, I pose these questions to my valued reader: Should not marijuana be placed in a higher Schedule than at present? Should it perhaps be *left off* the Schedules entirely, as it is with alcohol and tobacco? Should it not be decriminalized? Should it not be fully legalized? You be the judge. Perhaps after reading this *entire* book you will have the knowledge and understanding to re-assess your opinion.

Let us look again at some verifiable statistics:

DEATHS EACH YEAR:

- Tobacco   435,000
- Alcohol   85,000
- Prescribed Drugs   32,000
- Illicit drugs   17,000
- OTC drugs   8,000
- **MARIJUANA**   **000,000**

This is why our society must demand an end to the prohibition of this Amazing healing plant.

To those who have profited for years off of the misery and suffering of the sick and dying by maintaining the outright lie that marijuana should be a Schedule I with no redeeming qualities I say: "You will eventually get what you richly deserve. You and your greedy organizations will ultimately be dismantled and sent to the garbage dump of history."

All of the above brings up an important question: How in GOD's name did all of the deadly prescription drugs in common use today ever pass the government's supposedly strict criteria for legalization? **How indeed.**

Anyone who has studied all of the available literature and reviewed a large sample of the studies that are well documented will come to the inescapable conclusion that the arguments for marijuana legalization far outweigh the arguments against. **WAKE UP AMERICA!!!**

CHAPTER 15
JUST ANECTDOTAL EVIDENCE?
THINK AGAIN!

Dr. Andrew Weil, Integrative Medicine Doctor & Author:
"As a medical doctor and botanist, my aim has always
been to filter out the cultural noise surrounding the genus
Cannabis and see it dispassionately: as a plant with
bioactivity in human beings that may have therapeutic
value. From this perspective, what can it offer us? As it
turns out, a great deal. After more than 70 years of
misinformation about this botanical remedy, I am
delighted that we are finally gaining a mature
understanding of its immense therapeutic potential."

The single biggest lie spread by the media today is that there
is **ONLY anecdotal evidence** documenting the value of
marijuana to successfully treat a wide variety of ailments.
The implication always is that no "real" scientific studies have
ever been conducted. **NOTHING COULD BE FURTHER
FROM THE TRUTH!** *NOTHING.*

It's just that the vast anti-marijuana coalition (Big Pharmas' big
dollars, tobacco and alcohol lobbyists, private prison lobbyists,
timber lobbyists, and the United States government) **would
prefer** *that you didn't know about positive clinical trials*. They
simply do not publicize the pro-marijuana scientific studies, so
the public simply and quite logically assumes they do not
exist. **They do exist.** And they are quite easy to research.

It is most often said accusingly that marijuana leads to more
serious drug addictions, that marijuana is a "gateway drug".
As long ago as 1944 New York City Mayor Fiorello La Guardia

commissioned a study that lasted six years. It was conducted by the prestigious New York Academy of Medicine.

Their conclusion: "The use of marijuana does not lead to morphine or heroin or cocaine addiction". Many similar studies in subsequent years came to exactly the same conclusion.

Because of the increasing popularity and use of marijuana from its prohibition in 1937 through the '60s in spite of its illegal status, President Nixon created the Shafer Commission to study marijuana. Their unexpected report, *Marihuana: A Signal of Misunderstanding* contained a strong recommendation for decriminalization!

Nixon was outraged, and declared his fervent "War On Drugs", thereby creating the federal anti-marijuana policy which continues to this day.

A fifteen-month *federal* study released in 1982, conducted by the Institute of Medicine of the National Academy of Sciences concluded: "There is no evidence to support the belief that the use of one drug will inevitably lead to the use of any other drug". So much for marijuana being a "gateway drug".

It is often cited by the anti-marijuana lobby that smoking marijuana is at least as bad as smoking tobacco. Maybe worse. In 2006 a Dr. Tishkin of the University of California conducted a large scientific study that concluded that smoking marijuana, even heavily and regularly, does *not* lead to lung cancer.

Dr. Tishkin is quoted as reporting: "We hypothesized that there would be a positive correlation between marijuana use and lung cancer, and that the association would be more positive with heavier use. What we found was no association at all, and even a suggestion of some *protective effect*."

When have you ever read about THAT study in a newspaper? Never!

Researchers at the University of Virginia in the mid-1970s were the *first* to suggest the *protective* value of marijuana smoking. The United States government conducted *secret* research twenty years later hoping to disprove those results. Instead the research confirmed them! Needless to say this study was buried and never widely reported to this day.

In 2003 FIVE DIFFERENT SCIENTIFIC JOURNALS published articles indicating that cannabinoids were potential anti-cancer agents. **Every major newspaper ignored the stories.**

In 2009 the prestigious scientific journal *Cancer Prevention* reported that lifetime marijuana use is associated with significantly *reduced* risk of head and neck skin cancers. Any reporters pick up on this? Nope. Surprised?

I could go on and on. There have been over *thirty* carefully controlled peer-reviewed studies of marijuana use as it relates to various diseases. These maladies included AIDS, ALS, MS, PTSD and many others. (See Chapter 17.) Any diligent internet search can easily locate these studies.

The evidence is clear: the use of marijuana is harmless, it cannot kill you, it does not lead to other drug addictions, and it is proven to be of great medicinal value in a wide range of illnesses.

Yet in spite of this scientific evidence, (***not to mention 5,000+ years of rhetorical evidence)*** there are still many who are totally opposed to the legalization movement. This is mostly out of *pure ignorance of the truth,* and a reliance on misleading media reports and government propaganda fueled by an assortment of lobbyists' money.

Whether you realize it or not, the marijuana legalization movement continues to gain momentum. Is marijuana legalization unstoppable? Over the past two decades, 24 states have legalized marijuana for medical use, while five venues, four states (Alaska, Colorado, Oregon & Washington) and Washington, D.C. have legalized the purchase of recreational marijuana! (See Appendix III) We're winning, slowly.

The American public itself has begun to turn the tide in favor of legalization. National polls from Gallup, Pew Research, and the General Social Survey all show that a little over 50% of respondents support legalizing the drug for purely recreational pleasure. Polls also show that over 80% support medicinal use.

It is not just the public who wants to see marijuana's reach expand. Many states have dollar signs in their eyes when thinking about marijuana. Tax revenue generated from marijuana can go a long way toward supporting underfunded budgets. For instance, Colorado's education system alone may wind up receiving $40 million yearly from their marijuana tax revenue.

Of course, marijuana's hurdles are many, and greater expansion of legalization is far from a given. Among the challenges for the marijuana industry are the studies conducted that suggest marijuana is *in fact* a dangerous drug. A number of these studies have come to the conclusion that marijuana can cause cognitive or memory decline in regular users. Are they valid studies? Read Chapter 28 and decide.

Entirely New subject: **Are you fat?** You might consider trying the "marijuana diet"! The most common understanding is that marijuana gives individuals "the munchies". As such the expected findings from a scientific study would be that marijuana users should have higher BMIs (Body Mass Indices) and higher fasting insulin levels than non-users.

Surprisingly the results of a recent scientific study *contradict* this popular "given"! Investigators from the Conference of Quebec University Health Centers studied 786 adults age 18 to 74. They concluded that if there was any correlation between persons who use marijuana and those who don't as it relates to body mass index (BMI) and insulin levels **it favored marijuana use!**

A study published later in the research journal *Obesity* **confirmed** these results. The data showed that regular marijuana users had a BMI of 26.8 compared to non-users who had a BMI of 28.6. This was after researchers controlled for age, gender, and other important factors.

But, the observed benefits transcended only the users' BMIs. Marijuana users in the study also had lower fasting insulin and lower HOMA-IR, a measure of insulin resistance. These results were confirmed by yet another **study** published in *The American Journal of Medicine* suggesting marijuana may actually be effective in controlling Type 2 diabetes! Based on the findings, the study's authors came to this intriguing conclusion (*never* reported in the general media):

"The inverse association between marijuana use and BMI, fasting insulin, and HOMA-IR observed in our work supports evidence from a larger population of previous cross-sectional and follow-up investigations. As a result, cannabinoids from marijuana may be viewed as an interesting avenue for research on obesity and associated conditions."

Not only might marijuana help you lose weight, it might help you to quit smoking tobacco! A group of researchers from the University College in London, England, did a double blind study showing that a group of smokers given cannabidiol (CBD) had "a significant reduction in the number of tobacco cigarettes smoked, without increasing cravings". This study could piss off <u>BOTH</u> Big Pharma *and* Big Tobacco!

Over the past many decades widely publicized studies were specifically designed to prove conclusively that marijuana is bad in one way or the other. This was the *basic premise* of the studies at the<u> outset</u> . In the past five years, the focus has shifted.

Most studies, and there are thousands now in progress, are now set up to demonstrate the *benefits* of marijuana, not its imagined shortcomings. <u>*Medicinal efficacy* is now the primary focus of most new studies.</u>

For many decades there has been a perception, based on absolutely nothing factual, that long term marijuana use makes one stupid.

Personally I know two CEOs of significant-size exchange-listed companies who have smoked marijuana heavily and daily since the 1960s. Guess what? Amazingly they are not slobbering fools who can barely dress themselves. They are, in fact, highly articulate business persons with tack-sharp minds who frequently deliver eloquent public speeches!

Nor would anyone consider the many prominent public personalities mentioned after each Chapter heading in this book to fit the category of "stupid". They are anything but.

Is there even one study that put this stupidity nonsense to rest once and for all. The answer is: **"<u>YES!</u>"** A lengthy study of almost a thousand pairs of teenage *twins*, biologically-similar pairings for the closest possible control, showed absolutely no decline in IQ although one twin abstained completely and the other smoked marijuana regularly year after year after year. This result was consistent with many other non-sibling studies that have been performed for decades, but are seldom if ever reported in the media.

As soon as it is _widely accepted_ that long-term smoking of marijuana does not make one less intelligent and thereby less useful to society it will be a giant stepping stone towards the goal of universal legalization.

Back in 2009 the prestigious _Journal of Opioid Management_ published a landmark article, of course as always totally ignored by the media.   Dr. Sunil Aggarwal of the University of Washington and his colleagues researched _all_ of the controlled scientific clinical trials that had been conducted on marijuana between 1971 and 2009.

All of these studies confirmed conclusively that marijuana is a safe, effective medicine useful for specific medical conditions!

Dr. Aggarwal stated that: "Nearly all of the 33 published controlled clinical trials conducted in the United States have shown significant and _measurable_ benefits in subjects receiving the treatment."

He went on to say: **"The most common misconception among doctors and the general public regarding medical marijuana is that its effectiveness claims are substantiated only by compelling anecdotes from patients. What is not acknowledged is that 33 separate clinical trials with patients have been conducted and published in the United States by investigators at major research centers."**

Since 2009, as the march towards legalization picks up

speed, there have been hundreds more studies worldwide, all coming to exactly the same conclusions. Marijuana is safe. Marijuana is effective medicine. **Marijuana should be decriminalized and legalized. <u>Wake up America!</u>**

Possibly the most promising research, much of it in Israel, is showing that marijuana's CBD component has a potent anti-cancer-tumor effect. Studies done at the California Pacific Medical Center in San Francisco by Dr. Sean McAllister indicate that CBD depresses a gene known as ID-1. This gene is implicated in several types of aggressive cancers.

A study published in the prestigious *Journal of Neuroscience* showed that cannabidiol (CBD) helps prevent heroin cravings and withdrawal relapses by lowering the stimulus cue-induced heroin seeking impulses.

OK, so I'm an evil conspiracy theorist who believes that extra-terrestrials live among us and big Pharma hates marijuana. Let's discard the premise that there could be any number of possible clinical trial negative- influences proven, and assume that a TOTALLY honest and objective clinical trial is actually possible. How could such a trial be conducted?

The big question then is: <u>"What strain of marijuana will be used in the trials?"</u> (Or worse: "Will some 'standardized' synthetic cannabinoid from Big Pharma be used in the trial"?) Also, you must know:

1. Who is actually *funding* the trial?

2. Once you know the answer to "Who is funding?" ask: Who has ANY influence *over* the funding project itself, and over its results?

Just to weaken the possible value of clinical trials further, what delivery method will be used? Smoking (joints), vaping, sub-lingual (tinctures) or ingesting (e.g., brownies). <u>Each of these will show different effects for any one individual user to another from any given strain of marijuana.</u>

The fact is that, at best, clinical trials will simply delay legalization for decades, if not forever. With 5,000+ years of irrefutable evidence from millions of marijuana users, what exactly can any new *trial* on a <u>single strain or single chemical</u> possibly prove? Positive or negative, what real **usable** information can be gained. Answer: **NONE.**

The government has permitted the University of Mississippi to grow a carefully monitored "single clinical-trial" strain of marijuana for many years. Great! Except that, in fact , there are literally <u>thousands</u> of known and named different strains of marijuana. Chemically, there are literally millions of chemical component differences between them.

I have read that the particular strain being grown at Ole Miss is far from the best or most typical strain that they could be growing. In fact, it is apparently of rather poor quality. Why would THIS particular strain be the ONLY one approved for any new "scientific" tests? Why indeed.

In different strains there are differences in the presence (or lack thereof) of dozens of specific identifiable chemical components. There are differences in the relative proportions of whichever different chemicals happen to be present. There are differences in the percentages of any individual chemical that actually *is* present. The possible combinations considering the thousands of known marijuana strains are literally ***infinite***!

An important, and under-reported (Read: "suppressed by Big

Pharma") double-blind placebo-controlled study of people living with HIV/AIDS for at least six years demonstrated that marijuana can reduce neuropathic pain and promote weight gain without immunological compromises. This study was conducted by researchers at the University of California, San Francisco.

Two separate equally rigorous trials conducted by the University of California Center for Medicinal Cannabis Research (CMCR) demonstrated that smoked marijuana is highly effective in treating peripheral neuropathy.

Additional rigorous scientific trials have shown that marijuana can relieve neuropathic pain associated with multiple sclerosis and various neuropathies associated with trauma, vascular problems and herpes. In fact, any deep search of the internet could keep you busy for months, and could fill the pages of a dozen books far longer than this one.

You simply do not hear about these studies through conventional media. You never will.

For anyone who wants to acquire a thorough knowledge of marijuana use worldwide throughout the ages I strongly suggest reading the incredibly well researched book *Marijuana Medicine* by Christian Ratsch. It is published by the Healing Arts Press, Rochester, Vermont. It should be required reading for everyone who questions the absolute truth that marijuana is a powerful and totally safe medicine.

I cannot begin in this book to cover even a tiny fraction of the non-rhetorical scientific clinical studies of marijuana. The National Organization for the Reform of Marijuana Laws (NORML) recently made available its comprehensive booklet: *Emerging Clinical Applications for Cannabis and*

Cannabinoids: A Review of the Recent Scientific Literature. (Check out norml.org.) To read it is to be convinced.

You might also research the incredible work of Alison Myrden, "Granny Storm Crow", at beyondchronic.com. She documents literally hundreds of scientific marijuana studies. For an excellent, long but only partial list of published scientific studies, over two hundred of them, see: *"The Pot Book"*, edited by Dr. Julie Holland. It is available on Amazon.

If rhetorical "non-scientific" evidence is of interest to you, I suggest checking out a book by Joan Bello: *"The Benefits of Marijuana – Physical, Psychological and Spiritual"*. It contains about a hundred actual marijuana users' sworn testimonials.

So, do we NEED **more** marijuana studies? Well, more studies can't hurt. But to hear the constant litany: "We have to study the effects of marijuana before we can legalize it" is just abjectly absurd. It **HAS** been studied, rigorously and scientifically, for decades. All new studies can possibly accomplish short-term is more unjustified delay.

That Big Pharma and the media has managed to keep this information essentially unknown by the general public, most doctors, and almost all politicians, is testimony to the power of lobbying dollars. **A true National Disgrace.**

The key fact, as any marijuana user knows, is that it takes **PERSONAL EXPERIMENTATION** , self-conducted "clinical trials" if you wish, to find the strains that work best for a given individual's medical needs. It has taken me years of trying different strains and different delivery methods to arrive at a combination that works best for me and my MS symptoms.

Could there be something else, some better marijuana strain for me, out there? Of course there could! I couldn't possibly experiment with all but a small fraction of available strains. I have used some that do not work **AT ALL**. I have found some that have unwanted side-effects, such as excess sleepiness. I have found some that **solve** my various issues with **no** apparent side effects at all! It took time and effort.

NO CLINICAL TRIAL EVER DEVELOPED OR TO BE DEVELOPED COULD POSSIBLY HAVE LED ME TO MY CHOSEN MARIJUANA PRODUCTS. It is this fact alone that makes the entire matter of "we need years of scientific clinical trials" a waste breath.

Ever more clinical trials sound like a great idea. Clinical trials themselves are a great idea. In the context of "We Need Legalization **Now** To Relieve The Suffering Of Millions", all that more and more clinical trials can possibly accomplish, at best is to delay legalization perhaps indefinitely. At worst, if Big Pharma and others prevail, they will manage to "prove" that legalization is a mistake. (Take note of Chapter 28.)

FORGET UNNECESSARY WAITING FOR ENDLESS TRIAL RESULTS. IT IS A HOAX! *IN THE INTEREST OF HUMAN COMPASSION DECRIMINALIZE AND LEGALIZE NOW!*

In our age of capitalism, and of special interest lobby groups with almost limitless funds, one can only marvel at the crushing power of greed and avarice in the face of human need and suffering. Legalization of marijuana is a battle we must, and eventually will, win.

Only constant pressure on our public officials at all levels by a _truly informed and educated public_ can carry the day.

If you wish to support our cause in any way possible you can donate any amount on our extremely secure encrypted website at: TNWLF.org (The National Weed Legalization Fund) and get our free newsletter. Thanks!

CHAPTER 16
PTSD – OUR NATIONAL DISGRACE

SHAME ON THE USA

Froma Harrop, Syndicated Columnist:
"If drugs were legalized, narco-terrorists (including the Taliban) would lose their chief source of funds, drug gangs would go out of business, and the drug-fueled bloodbath now tormenting Mexico would end. Border security would vastly tighten as drug traffic dried up. Ending the war on drugs has support across the political spectrum. Many on the left regard America's drug laws as an assault on personal freedom and racist in their application. Prominent voices on the right -- for example, William F. Buckley and Milton Friedman -- long ago declared the war on drugs simply a dismal failure."

In July 2015 the excellent monthly magazine *THE AMERICAN LEGION MAGAZINE* ran a well-balanced article titled: *"The Cannabis Question"* by a contributor named Ken Olson. In part his article examined the case of a Marine Iraq veteran named Ryan who suffers from Post-Traumatic Stress Disorder (PTSD).

Speaking about the time after his return from combat, Ryan's mother is quoted as saying: "It was an absolute living hell after he managed to wreck two trucks, was jailed, disappeared for weeks at a time, and tried several times to commit suicide."

Ryan's nightmare continued for five long years, while taking the government's noxious cocktail of "narcotic painkillers, antidepressants, anti-anxiety medications, and sleeping pills, prescribed first by the military and then by the VA, which made him violent and unpredictable", says his mom.

Is Ryan's an isolated case? Not in my personal experience.
My next door neighbor has PTSD. He is under intense drug
treatment at a Tucson VA hospital. He tells me he has no
fewer than eight different deadly pills he takes twice daily. He
claims he is *totally* addicted to them. He talks openly about
turning his .45 pistol over and over in his hands at night,
deciding whether or not to endure another drugged-out
sleepless night. He says his VA psychologist (psychiatrist?)
knows all about this, and is "sympathetic".

His local-area past- reputation is one of violence and hostility
towards everyone. Fundamentally he is a very intelligent,
very decent guy, but I am absolutely convinced that
someday he will actually either kill himself, or perhaps kill
someone else.

I am an Army veteran myself, and belong to a local American
Legion Post. Thankfully I do not suffer from PTSD. I do use
marijuana to alleviate my multiple sclerosis symptoms. I hear
story after story after story of local PTSD patients in the same
general mental state as my neighbor. It has been an
unnecessary tragedy for decades. SHAME ON THE UNITED
STATES.

But what of Ryan? Well, he was fortunate enough to be living
in Maine, a marijuana-legal state.   There he found a rare
enlightened physician who prescribed marijuana to replace
the VA's noxious drug cocktail.   "Medical marijuana saved my
son's life", says his mom. Ryan himself says: "Now I'm in a
position physically and mentally where I can help other vets."
Merciful, happy ending.

Is Ryan's an isolated case? Hardly. Most veterans seek help at their local VA Hospital. The "help" they get has been limited to a deadly and addictive cocktail of opiates and anti-depressants. Most vets never get off this regimen. Over time the daily effects diminish, so they must take higher dosages or different drugs. It is an endless addicting cycle.

Up to 30% of all returning vets from Iraq and Afghanistan suffer from PTSD. It was known as "shell shock" in WWII & "battle fatigue" in WWI. Same ailment, different names.

In order to mollify legalization proponents there is always "legislation afoot" that, if passed, would clear the way for "clinical trials" of marijuana. They seldom materialize. When they do, all they accomplish is the *intended* endless delay.

PTSD affects different vets in different ways, some more severely than others. It is estimated that there are over twenty-three million veterans alive today. Hundreds of thousands, if not millions, suffer from PTSD. Unless you know a PTSD sufferer well personally you can never quite understand the mental and physical torture with which they live every day of their lives.

It is widely reported that there are twenty-two veteran suicides a day in the United States. **A DAY.**   Worse, this does not encompass reports from every state, nor does it take into account "accidental deaths" which may well actually be suicides. The real figure is thought to be closer to **50 per day.**

How many of these deaths are PTSD related? Probably most. How many might be prevented if marijuana was readily available in every state to these veterans? Probably most.

How can any country whose finest and bravest fought for our

Liberty and paid a terrible physical and mental price literally condemn so many to, at best, a life of misery, at worst, premature death? **How do our politicians live with themselves? It's incomprehensible.**

Exactly how is PTSD clinically defined? "It is a severe, debilitating and long-standing psycho-physical dis-function with intense episodic eruptions that derive from terrorizing, de-humanizing, and traumatizing experiences that destabilize the entire organism."

PTSD has both a physical and mental component. There is a spiritual, life-affirming value that is compromised. It affects the manner in which a PTSD sufferer presents to the world, and the perception of everything around him or her. It is a deep wound created by one or more unspeakably horrific events which does not heal at the emotional level.

There is also an actual physical change in the brain itself. Marijuana therapy for PTSD is very specific, and the reason it is so effective is well documented. Marijuana affects the amygdala area of the brain in a well-understood manner relating to the body's natural cannabinoid system.

One of marijuana's most important characteristics is the rapid speed with which inhaled smoke acts. This makes it possible for any PTSD patient to quickly determine their needed dose to obtain a given level of relief.

I have spoken to doctors at Veteran's Administration hospitals. Their hands have been tied. They know that the insane poisonous and addictive cocktails of pain killers and anti-depressants (worth many **billions** of dollars to Big Pharma) that they regularly prescribe could be eliminated almost *entirely* through marijuana prescriptions.

They could not, until very recently, prescribe marijuana to their PTSD patients because they are federal employees and marijuana is federally illegal. **This is an unspeakable American tragedy. Shame on the USA. Shame on our complicit politicians.**

Even worse, in the states where marijuana *is* legal for medical purposes, should veterans take it upon themselves to obtain a "marijuana card" and self-medicate with marijuana outside of the VA purview , they are then treated far differently when they do seek help from the VA doctors.

As a VA representative recently put it put it: " The use of marijuana is inconsistent with treatment goals". What goals? Misery and suicide? **This is criminal government insanity.**

Even *if* UNBIASED (read: "not in some way influenced by drug company money") studies are even possible, the fact that there are literally thousands of different marijuana strains, each with potentially different clinical outcomes on different conditions, renders the study of a few "standard quality-controlled strains" a total joke.

All these studies accomplish, regardless of their outcome, is endless delay, and of course endless prescriptions for every noxious and dangerous drug imaginable, and endless profits for Big Pharma.

How many veterans will continue a lifetime of suffering needlessly, and how many will continue the rash of veteran suicides, while the proposed clinical trials inevitably drag on endlessly? Screw the drug companies who turn out pain killers and anti-depressants by the billions and earn obscene profits. They deserve to go bankrupt.

Screw the doctors they control through their propaganda

literature. **LEGALIZE MARIJUANA NOW!**

The great shame of our government is the **ABSOLUTE FACT** that marijuana can replace the ***billions* *of dollars*** of taxpayer money that Big Pharma earns from the untold billions of pills they supply to the VA Hospitals.

Why haven't VA doctors prescribed marijuana? Well, they have had the perfect "excuse". Because marijuana is federally illegal and they are federal employees they have been *forbidden* by law from offering it. So they cannot and do not.

THIS WAS TRUE UNTIL A PROVISION OF THE 2017 VA FUNDING BILL IN MAY 2016 CONTAINED A PROVISION THAT PROHIBITS VA DOCTORS FROM ENFORCING MARIJUANA PROHIBITION! THIS WILL BE TRUE ONLY IN STATES WHERE MEDICAL MARIJUANA IS OTHERWISE LEGAL.

Will this change anything? Will it make *any* difference? Time will tell. We can only hope so. <u>The VA doctors are no different from most other American doctors</u>. They are just as influenced by Big Pharma and their endless perks and propaganda, and the decades of media lies as any other doctor.

There is overwhelming anecdotal evidence from veterans who have found a way to obtain marijuana and weaned themselves off of the deadly VA drug cocktails. An internet search can find many very convincing personal stories by vets who have found the relief they craved for years and thumbed their noses at the feds.

One researcher is dedicating her life to our brave PTSD afflicted veterans. Dr. Sue Sisley of Arizona has been featured in a TV documentary and in most major newspapers for her important research.

She is the primary investigator for an FDA-approved randomized controlled study of whole-plant marijuana for treating PTSD. She has faced almost insurmountable obstacles over many years to be allowed to conduct her research. Through her persistence (and that of many other lobbyists) PTSD has recently been added as one of the ailments that qualify for an Arizona Medical Marijuana Card.

In PTSD patients there is some dis-function of the brain's natural cannabinoid receptors. Research has shown that our cannabinoid receptors have a special affinity for marijuana cannabinoids, even more so than for the body's *own* cannabinoids! By administering marijuana the cannabinoid mechanism is restored to a more normal operational mode with the result of alleviating PTSD symptoms.

It is important to note that PTSD is not unique to veterans. Thousands of American citizens are exposed to unspeakable horrors that can leave them disabled mentally for life.

To understand why the marijuana legalization process has progressed at a snail's pace for decades, one must realize *that any such study is subjected to a* **THREE *NON-CONCURRENT* APPROVALS PROCESS!**

In chronological order, the United States Department of Agriculture (USDA), The United States Public Health Service (USPHS) , and the Drug Enforcement Agency (DEA) must _all be in agreement_ for any study to advance! They do not work simultaneously. Each reviews the work of the former. Delay, delay, delay. Talk about bureaucracy! Truly classic.

In late April 2016 the DEA officially approved smoking marijuana as legitimate medical research! What took it so long? Well, better late than never. It is actually allowing a controlled scientific clinical trial relating to PTSD!

A $2.2 million Colorado grant will permit "The Multidisciplinary Association for Psychedelic Studies" (MAPS) to perform a clinical trial. As with all government trials in the past, I wonder if the trial will be set up to prove conclusively that marijuana does **not** help PTSD patients. (Please read Chapter 28.) Can we trust ANY government trial to be objective? Can we trust any trial *at all* to be objective? We shall see.

In this particular PTSD case, The USDA approved this study over FIVE YEARS AGO, in 2011 (**that's about 40,000 veteran suicides ago.**) This was followed THREE FULL YEARS LATER, in 2014, when the United States Public Health Service finally signed on. And then after another TWO YEARS, the DEA gave its blessing. GOD help us if we ever have to approve a study rapidly for something we really consider urgent!

Of course, whether MAPS is actually a *neutral* third party remains to be seen. Positive, scientific PTSD studies have been conducted for years *without* government blessing. Will MAPS be charged with the responsibility of *confirming* all of the positive results, or *refuting* them? Again, we'll see.

Finally, let me propose a nominee for "Government Disgrace of the Decade". We need look no further than United States Drug Enforcement Agency *Chief* Mr. Chuck Rosenberg. (Could he be related to Harry Anslinger?) Mr. Rosenberg has publically dismissed the *entire idea* of medical marijuana as **"a joke".**

Mr. Rosenberg is quoted as saying: "What really bothers me is the notion that marijuana is also medicinal.....which it is not.

If you talk about smoking the leaf of marijuana…..which is what most people are talking about when they talk about medicinal marijuana…..it has never been shown to be safe or effective as a medicine."

WHAT ROCK HAS THIS FOOL BEEN HIDING UNDER? HOW CAN ANYONE POSSIBLY BE THIS MISINFORMED? And this guy somehow became **HEAD OF THE DRUG ENFORCEMENT AGENCY? Was he chosen for that job on the basis of his absurd negative attitude towards marijuana? INCREDIBLE.**

America is in SO much trouble!

CHAPTER 17
MEDICAL CONDITIONS
AND MARIJUANA USE

Laura Ingraham, Syndicated Radio Host & Author:
"I think all of us have either gone through cancer or
family members, and it's a terribly painful disease. I think
you have a lot of sympathy. There's a lot of public
sympathy for medical marijuana use."

The University of Arizona publishes an interesting brochure
titled: "Using Medical Marijuana Safely". Much of the
information that follows was derived from that brochure. They
list the following uses of Medical Marijuana, as stated in
Arizona statute 36-2801:

- Cancer
- Glaucoma
- HIV
- AIDS
- Hepatitis C
- ALS (Lou Gehrig's Disease)
- Chohn's disease
- Agitation from Alzheimer's disease
- Any chronic or debilitating disease or medical condition
  that causes:

1. Cachexia or wasting syndrome;
2. Severe and chronic pain;
3. Severe nausea;
4. Seizures characteristic of epilepsy, or severe and
   persistent muscle spasms including those

characteristic of multiple sclerosis.

Recently, PTSD (Post Traumatic Stress Disorder) has been added to the Arizona list after some serious lobbying.

Marijuana Sativa strain genetics are generally associated with stimulating, uplifting or energizing effects on one's mental state. They can:
- Reduce depression
- Reduce pain awareness
- Reduce nausea
- Increase focus
- Increase creativity
- Relieve common headaches
- Relieve migraines
- Stimulate appetite

On the other hand, Marijuana **Indica** genetics are associated with:
- Aid in sleep
- Relaxation
- Calming effects
- Reduced inflammation
- Reduced pain
- Reduced inter-ocular pressure
- Stimulation of appetite
- Relief of common headaches
- Relief of migraines

As mentioned earlier, there is a website you must check out. A lady named Alsion Marden, who calls herself "Granny Storm Crow", documents studies of the medicinal effects of marijuana. She has set up the informative website URL: beyondchronic.com. It is well worth accessing.

Remember, Big Pharma has at least one prescription pill for each and every condition listed below. If you take the time to read the fine print included with these drugs you will almost always find one item listed under the contra-indications.
DEATH!

No one claims that marijuana CURES anything, any more than do most prescription pills actually *cure* anything. Some Israeli research has shown that marijuana might actually cure some cancers. Most important, no one can claim that marijuana has EVER killed anyone, because it has not.

Among the diseases that have seen positive relief in documented marijuana studies are:
- Acquired immune deficiency syndrome (AIDS)
- Attention Deficit Disorder (ADD)
- Attention Deficit Hyperactivity Disorder (ADHA)
- Alcoholism
- Amyotrophic lateral sclerosis (ALS, aka Lou Gehrig's Disease)
- Alzheimer's disease
- Anorexia
- Arthritis
- Asthma
- Atherosclerosis (hardening of the arteries)
- Autism
- Bipolar disorder
- Brain trauma
- Cancer

- Crohn's disease
- Cystic fibrosis
- Cystitis
- Depression
- Dermatitis
- Diabetes
- Distonia
- Eczema
- Edema
- Epilepsy
- Fibromyalgia
- Gastro-esophageal reflux disease (GERD)
- Glaucoma
- Hepatitis
- Herpes
- Human immunodeficiency virus (HIV)
- Huntington's disease
- Irritable bowel syndrome (IBS)
- Menopause
- Migraines
- Morning Sickness
- Methicillin-resistant staphylococcus aureus (MERS)
- Multiple sclerosis (MS)
- Muscular dystrophy
- Nausea
- Neuropathic pain
- Osteoporosis
- Pain
- Pancreatitis
- Parkinson's disease
- Post-Traumatic Stress Disorder (PTSD)
- Pruritus
- Restless leg syndrome
- Sickle cell disease

- Spasticity
- Spinal cord injury
- Stroke
- Tourette's syndrome
- Ulcerative colitis

The above is only a PARTIAL list of conditions for which using marijuana has been shown to relieve the pain and discomfort, and in certain conditions, actually cure the malady.

Add to this list the countless anecdotal accounts of marijuana's curative powers and no reasonably literate/average intelligence individual who takes the time **to actually research marijuana's positive values and become _truly informed_** can make any strong argument _against_ legalization. We discussed these contra-legalization arguments in Chapter 13.

Incredible as it may seem to some, there are active movements in states where medical marijuana is legal to have it available to elementary school nurses to administer to kids as needed! This has already happened in New Jersey, and by the time you read this it will likely be true in Colorado.

Just how does marijuana work its magic? Here, greatly oversimplified are the apparent physical mechanisms:

Our body has "CB1 receptors" that are prominent in the brain, and "CB2 receptors" that are prominent in the peripheral nervous system and the immune system.

Cannabidiol (CBD) does not _bind to_ the CB1 or CB2 receptors as does tetrahydrocannabinol (THC) or cannabinol (CBN). THC _stimulates_ the CB1 receptors; CBN _stimulates_ the CB2 receptors. CBD has a stimulating effect on _both_ the CB1 and

CB2 receptors. (Incidentally, CBN is not found in the marijuana plant itself. It is a breakdown product of THC.)

CBD also binds directly to the TRPV-1 receptor, which is known to mediate inflammation, pain perception, and body temperature.

CBD inhibits the breakdown of the body's own natural cannabinoid, "anandamide". It does this by suppressing the enzyme-fatty-acid amide hydroxylase, which breaks down anandamide. In this way CBD *preserves* the body's own natural cannabinoids. Who knew?

Another action of CBD is that it stimulates the release of another natural cannabinoid called 2-AG. CBD also powerfully *opposes* the action of the THC at the CB1 receptor, dulling THC's psychoactive effect. The higher the percentage of CBD in a product the lesser is the psychoactive effect from the THC present.

CBD also appears to directly activate the body's serotonin receptors causing an anti-depressant effect. This is one reason (of many) why it can be so valuable to our PTSD veterans.

Scientists at the Technion-Israel Institute of Technology in Haifa recently released the preliminary results of a cancer study that examined the effects of fifty varieties of marijuana with 200 *different* cancer cells. While it's still far too soon to draw any conclusions, their findings are reportedly cause for great optimism.

The researchers noticed that cannabinoids have the ability to slow tumor growth. They apparently can selectively promote cancer cell death by a process known as "apoptosis." These findings confirm those uncovered in a Spanish study from 2013 which specifically looked at THC as a potential anti-cancer agent. The scientists in Israel wondered how different combinations of marijuana derivatives, including the dose and delivery method, might affect different types of cancer cells.

Dr. David Mein, leader of the Israeli research team, stated: "There is a large body of scientific data which indicates that cannabinoids specifically inhibit cancer cell growth and promote cancer cell death. In addition to active cannabinoids, marijuana plants also contain a multitude of other therapeutic agents, such as terpenoids and flavonoids that are usually present in small quantities, but can have beneficial therapeutic effects, especially as synergistic compounds to cannabinoids."

Dr. Mein's specialized area of study is "cell cytoskeletons". This discipline specifically addresses the movement and division processes of cancerous cells. In search of compounds that influence cell structure Dr. Mein eventually arrived at marijuana. He was anxious to fill the void of knowledge surrounding it. He did!

Cancer patients have been prescribed and used medical marijuana for pain, nausea, and appetite loss associated with treatment. The growing body of evidence science has to offer makes one wonder what else *Marijuana – The Wonder Weed* is capable of achieving!

Let us for a moment put aside thousands of years of *anecdotal* evidence for the curative powers of marijuana. As a sufferer from multiple sclerosis and peripheral neuropathy myself, elsewhere in this book I tell my "anecdotal" story of the relief that I have achieved through marijuana use when all else has failed.

One of the problems about "scientific marijuana studies" over the years is that the basic purpose of each study at the outset has been to show the HARM marijuana was imagined to cause, *not* to investigate its benefits. The focus was always to prove the *harm* premise.

If one realizes that there are actually many deaths recorded in the United States every year FROM OVERDOSING ON PLAIN DRINKING WATER, than one can understand that, given a sufficient quantity of virtually *anything*, death <u>can</u> occur. Set up a study, dose a lab rat with enough "medicine", and voila! One dead rat. Proof positive. But of what?

In fact it is just such an experiment that is often cited by the mis-informed anti-marijuana crowd to prove conclusively that marijuana *can* kill. They force-fed a rat an amount of marijuana that was the equivalent of a human ingesting ten pounds of marijuana at once or smoking thousands of joints in a single day. Guess what? The rat died! Duh.

At least in humans, marijuana, even taken in excess, ***CANNOT* KILL!** There has never been one single documented case of death by a marijuana overdose in human history!

If marijuana can shrink tumors in mice and reduce the number of seizures a child suffers from hundreds a day to a few, it just may be the **"Wonder Drug of All Time"**!

Let's not forget, this miracle herb has been in the bong behind a zillion college dorm couches all along!

Who knew?

CHAPTER 18
SMOKE IT, EAT IT, VAPE IT,
OR RUB IT ON

Hugh Hefner, **Founder of the Playboy Empire:**
"I applaud the legalization of marijuana in Washington State. I've supported legalization since the 1960s."

There are many different ways to consume marijuana. Probably the most common is rolling the crushed buds in rolling papers and smoking as a cigarette (a "joint"). This has the disadvantage that one is consuming the burned paper which may contain harmful chemicals as well as the marijuana. Using special hemp-based rolling-paper eliminates this burnt-paper problem.

One can eliminate the uptake of ash, tar and toxins by smoking the crushed buds in a pipe made of some inert material such as glass. Some pipes, often referred to as "bongs" or "water pipes" use water to filter out much of the tar and ash while reducing the temperature of the smoke. In theory this reduces throat and lung irritation. Because this method allows a large volume of smoke to be inhaled at once, coughing fits can occur.

A popular method of marijuana use is the vaporizer. In principal this heats the marijuana enough to vaporize the active cannabinoids without actually burning the plant matter. Electric coils are employed so the plant material is exposed to no live flame.

There are also "marijuana e-cigarettes" similar to the vapor pens used by individuals who are trying to quit conventional tobacco smoking. These pen devices, which are battery operated, often contain oils or tinctures rather than plant matter. As is the case with many things that are working well, the government in "the public interest" is cracking down on the labeling of *all* e-cigarettes. What a surprise!

Another common method of using marijuana is tinctures, using glycerin or alcohol mixed together with finely powdered marijuana or marijuana oil. These are placed drop by drop under the tongue for rapid absorption.

It should be noted that the time it takes for marijuana to take effect varies depending on how it is consumed. It takes around five minutes for inhaled marijuana to begin to work its magic, and around a half hour for maximum effect. On the other hand, marijuana edibles take around forty-five minutes to begin to have an effect, and as long as three hours for the maximum effect to be achieved.

After the greatest effect is reached, depending upon the amount consumed the entire effect *wears off* after anywhere from thirty minutes to three hours. The fact that it takes so much longer for consumed edibles to reach maximum effect leads some new users to consume more and more of the edible thinking that the desired effect wasn't reached. This can lead to consuming far more than intended, with much longer lasting effects.

Although a fatal dose of marijuana is impossible, overdosing will invariably lead to "couchlock". You and your couch or bed become one! When I was new to marijuana I ate consecutive quarters of a marijuana dark chocolate bar within fifteen minutes. Who knew? I never gave the first quarter bar time to take effect. I was totally immobilized for hours!

If a person is new to using marijuana couchlock CAN be scary, albeit harmless. 911 time? It often is.

The fact is that everyone experiences the effect of marijuana differently. A particular strain might make one person sleepy, another not at all. One person might get great pain relief from a particular strain, while another achieves no relief at all.

Everyone needs to be be aware that the use of concentrates such as hash or wax or shatter will lead to much more pronounced effects than one gets from medical grade marijuana buds. It should also be noted that medical grade marijuana can be much stronger than common "street grade" marijuana.

There is a huge range of potency between different strains. Most dispensaries can show you a chart with the approximate potency of each strain they sell, based on lab analyses. The two most important constituents, psychoactive THC (tetrahydrocannabinol) and CBD (cannabidiol) usually make up about 90% of the analyses. There are also the important terpenes and about ten other components that are usually also listed. (In fact there are hundreds of   identifiable chemicals in marijuana.)

THE KEY IS TO USE JUST ENOUGH MARIJUANA TO GET THE DESIRED MEDICAL EFFECT WHILE MINIMIZING ANY SIDE EFFECTS. Generally this takes *a lot of experimentation.*

No doctor will *ever* be able to prescribe a specific quantity of a specific strain for a specific condition and have any idea whether it will be effective. This fact alone gives all doctors great hesitation when considering marijuana for a patient.

Ointments & salves are topical rubs that transfer active

cannabinoids from marijuana plant matter to a preparation that can be absorbed trans-dermally (i.e., through the skin.)

They react with cannabinoid receptors in the skin and help increase blood flow. Because they cannot reach the central nervous system through the skin they have no psychoactive or drowsy effects.

Safety is the primary benefit of all marijuana use. There is no overdose level. No one has ever died from ingesting too much marijuana, nor has marijuana ever caused liver or kidney damage or organ failure. This singles out marijuana from all prescribed pain medicines as not *only* being effective but **extremely harmless to the human body**.

In the name of compassion for all American citizens the federal government simply must reconsider ALL of its positions on marijuana as soon as possible.

CHAPTER 19
MARIJUANA EDIBLES –
BUYER BEWARE!

Juan Williams, Fox News Analyst & Columnist:
"I think we've had three decades of this war on drugs...
And what do we see? Is there any decrease in the people
who are selling drugs? My gosh, we have more people
selling drugs right now. We have more young people
doing drugs. We have more people in jail than anybody
else. And most of it's related to drug-related offenses.
Why is it that we shouldn't think about rehabilitation or
doing something differently? Chris Christie, a good
Republican, governor of New Jersey, just said the other
day, 'The war on drugs has been an absolute, abysmal
failure.' "

Marijuana consumed as edibles, as opposed to smoked,
vaped or in sublingual form, are available wherever marijuana
can be legally purchased. Often called "medibles", short for
"medicinal-edibles", they come in every imaginable yummy
form. Of course there are the ubiquitous brownies that have
been around for decades. (Thank you Alice B. Toklas!)

Today there are marijuana gum drops, lollypops, cookies,
cakes, hard candies, chocolate bars, shakes, soft drinks,
smoothies, you name it, someone is making it, and thousands
of Americans are legally consuming it.

Proponents of edible marijuana products claim quite correctly
that in theory ingesting marijuana should be safer than
smoking it. Although countless studies have shown that
smoking tobacco products is far more dangerous than
smoking marijuana, eating marijuana is in fact safer.

154

There is a problem with various edibles that has become evident as the many states where it is legal gain experience and collect data (not to mention collecting huge taxes). Getting the *correct dose* from an edible product can be very tricky for a number of reasons:

- Different strains of marijuana used in edibles can have different effects on different users. No two people sucking on the same marijuana-lollypop will get the exact same result. Of course this is true for using marijuana in *any* form. It is a *very* personal experience that requires months if not years of cautious experimentation to find what works best for any individual's ailment.

- The actual *amount* of the psychoactive chemicals present in any edible, as must be stated on the labels, has been shown in many lab tests to often be *very* inaccurate. It is most often lower than stated (not a big surprise, paying for something that one is not actually getting) but *can* be higher, sometimes much higher.

The problem with this "uncertainty scenario" is that, in an industry that needs as little *legitimate* negative-press as possible (it has gotten decades of totally-misleading illegitimate negative media coverage and government lies) the uncertainties about the potency of any given edible is very problematic.

I am a legal marijuana user. I suffer from painful leg neuropathy, as well as multiple sclerosis, and I get incredible relief from marijuana.   I have learned a lesson about edibles: If the label says: "Start slowly, try a bit at a time, and increase consumption once you know how this product affects you",

BELIEVE THE LABEL! If there is no such label, *pretend* there is! Case in point:

As I related earlier, I bought a rather small dark chocolate bar (my first ever- - I prefer brownies) that actually had a label statement similar to the above. I read the THC content and it was quite low. Because I had been consuming marijuana in other forms for years I had acquired a pretty good idea of a useful dose and what effect to expect from it.

So, instead of taking a small cautionary bite as the label suggested, I broke off one-quarter of the bar, which is where it was conveniently scored. It was truly delicious! Maybe the best dark chocolate bar ever! I continued to eat the whole yummy bar. Based on the labeled THC content its psychoactive effect should have been relatively minimal. Well, not exactly!

Within an hour or so (edibles take a while to enter the system) all I wanted to do was sleep! In fact, all I COULD do was sleep. I had what is referred to in marijuana slang as "couchlock". I literally spent the next six hours in a lovely but totally unproductive state of euphoria, drifting in and out of a state of near parlysis and deep sleep, which was NOT my intention (I normally work a solid fourteen-hour day.)

When I told a long-time stoner friend about the incident he almost wet his pants laughing! All I can say is be cautious with all medibles. If you happen to be a "newbie" with little or no marijuana experience, be ESPECIALLY cautious!

The point of this story is that whoever made that chocolate bar added FAR MORE marijuana to their recipe than was stated on the label. In fact, I'd guess at least ten times as much!

Perhaps they did it as a joke. Perhaps they were simply incompetent. This is one excellent argument for strict regulations pertaining to the actual marijuana content of each edible product.

What if I had eaten another bar right after the first? Would I be in any danger of a deadly overdose? No, because it is clinically *impossible* to die from an overdose of marijuana. The area of the brain that it affects does not control breathing. The only possible danger would have been if I rolled out of bed and broke my neck!

Of course if you make your own edibles, as many marijuana patients, including me, do, *you control* the amount of marijuana and THC present. In addition you can use specific strains that you have found to be effective for your particular ailment. There are at least twenty marijuana cookbooks available at Amazon! **Bon appetite'!**

IMPORTANT WARNING (restated from earlier in this book): Regardless of whether you consider marijuana to be harmful or not, or a "gateway drug" or not, **KEEP ALL FORMS, ESPECIALLY YUMMY EDIBLE FORMS, OUT OF THE REACH OF CHILDREN AND TEENS!**

Whether it is raw buds and leaves or brownies, cookies, lollypops, a smoothie or whatever these items MUST be treated as edibles **for adult use only.** You manage to keep truly deadly substance out of their reach...drain cleaners, insecticides, rat poison, and over-the-counter and prescription drugs...**PLEASE** be equally diligent about ALL forms of marijuana.

CHAPTER 20
CHOOSE YOUR STRAIN

Roseanne Barr, **Actress & Comedian:**
"Does anybody doubt that controlling and taxing pot would bring billions and billions of dollars endlessly streaming into our national wallet? As things stand now, two things are happening: 1. Tens of millions of Americans buy marijuana, and 2. Many essential social and educational programs are on life-support if not dead already, for lack of funding. Hello? The Marijuana market is not going away, so why not turn this to our advantage and steer the steady revenue into places that would help make life better for most Americans?"

The personal use of marijuana is far more complex an issue than most imagine. The three key variables are:

1. Which strain to use;
2. How to use it;
3. How much to use.

These variables are fundamental to the entire industry.   It is **impossible** to determine these for any individual person through clinical tests and trials. There are simply too many variables. Only by long-term personal *trial and error* can the optimum consumption variable-set for any individual's needs be determined.

Everyone feels the effects of marijuana differently. No two individuals ingesting the identical product in the identical way are likely to get the same effect.

Using identical products one might person might get sleepy, another not. One individual might feel profound pain relief, while another, with similar pain, might get no relief at all. It is a fact that different individuals react differently to a given strain. At this writing there are well over a thousand distinctly different named and analyzed marijuana strains.

The goal of any user is to achieve the desired effect while minimizing any possible side effects. This can take months, if not years, of personal trial and error.

Can marijuana EVER be studied objectively? Unfortunately the answer is "NO", and this may be the #1 obstacle to marijuana legalization. The government wants to achieve standardization. It can *never* achieve it.

The exact same marijuana strain grown by two different growers from seed from the same female plant will produce similar but *noticeably different* results. Whether it is grown in soil or hydroponically, whether it is fertilized naturally (think bat guano) or chemically, and even the individual farmers growing, harvesting and drying "styles" all produce a different product. The fact is, NO TWO MARIJUANA BUDS ARE ALIKE!

When the government finally allows wide-spread testing, it will be with the one "standardized" strain being grown at the University of Mississippi. This is but one of over a thousand different readily available strains! What could these government tests possibly prove? Not much.

What it could cause is years of delay in the implementation of legalization. There will NEVER be enough "conclusive medical data" to satisfy the government. Big Pharma will be certain to see to that. Delay is inevitable.

With literally hundreds of different strains, pure Indicas, pure Sativas, intra-Sativa or intra-Indica crosses, or hybrid Indica-Sativa crosses (and even breed in some Ruderalis-marijuana) there are virtually limitless possible strains. More new strains are created every day.

Contrary to what some dispensaries will pitch to marijuana patients, every single marijuana strain affects every individual differently. This is why "scientific research" is worthless for all practical purposes. It is impossible to test every strain variant for every human disease. There are simply too many strains and too many diseases, and too many different physiologies.

One only need study the chemical analyses sheets available at the dispensary for those twenty or so strains they happen to sell to recognize the VAST DIFFERENCES between the amounts of chemical components present in each strain.

Every patient needs to experiment and continue to experiment in order to determine which strain is best for alleviating their particular symptoms.

The ultimate goal for any patient is ***symptom relief.*** All any patient really ever requires (and in fact all they will ever get) is solid anecdotal evidence from users with similar conditions. Most dispensaries can at least offer some guidance in this direction. No doctor can or will.

It could be decades, if ever, before an enlightened physician will have collected enough anecdotal evidence to advise, with even *some* certainty, that a particular strain or group of strains would be a good starting point for a given patient's healing experimental adventure.

When we are considering *recreational* marijuana use finding the "right" strain for whatever effect you are striving is MUCH easier. A high is a high! The need to find THE strain to relieve your unique medical symptoms is much harder.

There are any number of wonderful books in print available

on Amazon that list hundreds of strains by name and give good advice on the taste, aftertaste, strength, and every imaginable effect one can expect from each of them. You might still want to experiment, but your choices will be narrowed by your thorough research of the details reported by thousands of recreational users.

Once you have acquired your marijuana in whatever form you choose, you must learn how to preserve it. It can lose potency rather quickly if not properly stored.

To preserve marijuana flowers and plant material from deterioration, store in a dark, cool place in an airtight rigid container. For less than 90 days, storage below 50 degrees F and 55% humidity is considered optimal.

For longer storage, store marijuana in a freezer below 4 degrees F. Never thaw and refreeze marijuana, and never subject it to greater than 80 degrees F such as found in a hot car or glove compartment. Never try to rehydrate dry marijuana as all this does is encourage mold and bacteria to flourish.

Pressed hashish can be stored indefinitely in a freezer in a vacuum-sealed food storage bag. Store tinctures in the refrigerator. Shake tinctures vigorously for each use as the marijuana can precipitate out and/or attach to the walls of the dropper bottle. Oils and waxes are the most concentrated forms of medical marijuana with THC as high as 80%. It is best to freeze these in *single-use* packages.

All forms of marijuana edibles are best frozen and thawed out as needed. It is a good idea to package the amounts you plan to consume at one time in individual zip-lock freezer bags.

Adherence to the above guidelines will insure that your stash will always have the potency it had when you acquired it.

CHAPTER 21
DO WORDS MATTER?

Willie Nelson, Grammy Award-Winning Musician:
"I think eventually, the worse the economy gets, the more sense it makes to legalize marijuana. First of all, you save all that money being spent on drug enforcement, all the money that goes for putting people in prison for smoking pot. There's just millions and millions of dollars that can be saved by legalizing it. All the people who grow for the drug cartels in Mexico and the cartels all over the rest of the world, they don't want to see it legalized."

I am convinced that the very *names* of many marijuana strains are a detriment to legalization. They just sound too scary or creepy! They certainly do not sound "scientific"!

Much of the crossbreeding to produce hybrid strains has been done within the counter-culture. As such, and without thought of legalization for medical purposes or otherwise, we have ended up with an assortment of fantasy names that sound like anything *but* serious medicine.

Among today's most popular strains are:

- Acid (with absolutely no connection to the street drug LSD)
- AK-47
- Amsterdam Cheese
- Atomic Haze
- Bubblegum
- Chem Dawg
- Chronic
- Cripple Creek

- Deadhead
- Granddaddy Purple
- Great White Shark
- Green Crack (again, no connection whatsoever to any street drug)
- Hog
- Jack Flash
- L.A. Confidential
- LSD (a strain that has absolutely nothing to do with the drug LSD)
- Ménage-A-Trois
- Nebula
- NYC Diesel
- Quasar
- Rock Star
- Russian Rocket Fuel
- Skunk
- ThaiTanic
- Trainwreck
- Wappa
- Yoda

And there are hundreds more names that are equally weird!

Now I ask, can you in your wildest dreams imagine any physician actually prescribing any of the above strains for any ailment, even if it was proven beyond a shadow of doubt to be the *correct* strain? I think not.

Doctor to patient: "I think some AK-47 would greatly relieve your MS symptoms."

Doctor to patient: "For your serious PTSD I think a Trainwreck would be ideal."

Doctor to patient : "I know your chemo is nauseating you. I can help relieve that with some Bubblegum."

Doctor to patient: "Let's try Yoda first, and if you don't get pain relief from that I think a Ménage-A-Trois would be in order".

Pick any name above and any disease and I cannot imagine any doctor at any time in the future writing that strain on a prescription!

Strains such as the above are common and popular today. There are hundreds of others with equally ridiculous names (Purple Urkel comes quickly to mind. Matanuska Thunderfuck isn't far behind!) Unfortunately, seeing these strains in one's legal dispensary and considering them as serious medicine is a bit unnerving to say the least!

Even the less fantastic popular strain names don't exactly reek of serious medicinal potential: Ambrosia; Blackberry; Blueberry; Cheese Cake; Grapefruit; Ice Cream; Juicy Fruit; Mango; Papaya; Pineapple; Sour Cream, and Watermelon. This sounds more like a grocery list than a list of potent serious medicines!

Aside from doctor's prescriptions, I have a hard time imagining the published scientific paper of a double-blind study of "Skunk" being taken very seriously!

Big Pharma makes up ridiculous names for their products but at least they "sound" grounded in science as opposed to fantasy. Prescription names such as "Satavix", Epidolex and "Marinol" seem far more appropriate for a medicine than "Russian Rocket Fuel"!

Words DO matter.

CHAPTER 22
CONCLUSIVE PROOF
THAT MARIJUANA KILLS

**Milton Friedman, Recipient of the Nobel Prize in
Economics:**
**"There is no logical basis for the prohibition of
marijuana...$7.7 billion [spent on prohibition's
enforcement] is a lot of money, but that is one of the
lesser evils. Our failure to successfully enforce these
laws is responsible for the deaths of thousands of people
in Colombia. I haven't even included the harm to young
people. It's absolutely disgraceful to think of picking up a
22-year-old for smoking pot. More disgraceful is the
denial of marijuana for medical purposes."**

I thought I'd post this Chapter headline before the anti-
legalization media gets around to it! You see, the headline is
absolutely *true*.....it just leaves out some important details, a
very common problem in marijuana journalism and
government propaganda.

A very interesting scientific United States Government study
was presented to the United States Congress by Raymond P.
Shafer on March 22nd, 1972 . **What was described in
painful (for the monkeys and dogs involved) detail was
their horrible and almost instant deaths from direct
intravenous injections of massive doses of pure THC
extract (tetrahydrocannabinol), the psychoactive
ingredient in marijuana.**

It was eventually deduced that the deaths that occurred were
due to the insolubility of pure THC in blood. It precipitated
out and clogged blood vessels. THC is fat soluble, not water

soluble, and cannot be injected without killing the patient .

If the anti-marijuana media picks up on this study, the great revelation of "why?" would end there. **Marijuana kills!** Proof positive. End of story. Period.

The presentation to Congress went on to say that they then used tinctures (THC mixed with various carriers such as glycerin and alcohol) orally, and came to the following conclusions: "In summary, _enormous_ (emphasis mine) doses of _tetrahydrocannabinol_, and all _tetrahydrocannabinol_ concentrated extracts ingested orally were unable to produce death or organ pathology in monkeys and dogs."

"It did, however, produce fatalities in small rodents due to profound central nervous system depression. Proposed media headline: "Oral doses of marijuana kills rats." **Marijuana kills!** Proof positive. End of story. Period.

The _non_-lethal oral consumption of 3g/kg of tetrahydrocannabinol by a dog and a monkey (the actual amounts they were fed) would be comparable to a 154-pound human eating approximately forty-six pounds, 21kg, of one-percent THC marijuana, or ten-pounds of five-percent hashish, at one time.

These doses would be comparable to a 154-pound human _smoking_ at one time almost three pounds of one-percent THC marijuana, 250,000 times the usual smoked dose. This is over _a million times_ the minimal effective dose, assuming fifty-percent destruction of the THC by combustion. Hello! Anyone you know planning on consuming forty-six pounds of marijuana at a sitting? Or smoking three pounds of marijuana consecutively? I think not.

<u>INTERESTING OBSERVATION</u>: It is a fact that pure plain drinking water consumed in excess can actually kill. There are dozens of deaths reported annually from water overdoses, generally by rapidly rehydrating athletes. Not one single death has EVER occurred in all of human history from a marijuana overdose!

Reasonable conclusion: Consuming marijuana is actually safer than drinking water!

I don't believe I have ever seen *that* headline in the media.

CHAPTER 23
THE KILLER DRUGS KIDS TAKE TODAY

Peter Baume, Former Australian Minister for Health, Minister for Education & Minister for Aboriginal Affairs: "Many people who think of themselves as the beneficiaries of prohibition are really net losers. Parents are much more at risk of losing their children under prohibition than they would be if there was some kind of system where we had some measure of control over illicit drugs."

The United States "War On Drugs" has been, by any definition, an abysmal failure. Billions of dollars of taxpayer money has been wasted on a "War" that has been lost, year in and year out. The cartel criminals clearly prevail. Street drugs have become more popular and available year after year after year. Deaths have gone up year after year after year. **Wake up America!**

The biggest concern about marijuana legalization has always been the damage it allegedly might do to American youths.

As controversial as the following statement may be: *"I am certain that if marijuana was actually as readily available to kids as street drugs are today, and as inexpensive, and they were taught the <u>real</u> dangers of other street drugs, that they would not be killing themselves and irreparably damaging their organs with all of the readily available deadly poisons they currently buy and use. They would stay with marijuana"*.

The marijuana high is so very pleasant and fulfilling it is inconceivable to me that any marijuana user would ever even think of turning to street drugs. It just would not happen. It is the people who have never even *tried* recreational marijuana, and have not the least clue about what a wonderful experience marijuana can be, who are the biggest doubters. To them I say: **"Try it, you'll like it!"**

Fortunately, in the latest polls over 50% of all Americans support full recreational legalization. Fully 90% have finally realized that medical marijuana is an absolute no brainer. **Shame on our federal government.**

Marijuana has never killed anyone. An overdose is impossible. Most users simply chill out or pass out. They don't die! They cannot die. And the effect only lasts from four to six hours.

Any of the drugs listed below can be bought by any pre-teen or teen who makes even a modest effort to find it. I don't care if it is in an affluent city, a ghetto, or a farm community, these drugs can be bought *everywhere.* Some can even be bought over the counter or on line!

The basic problem is that corrupt, sophisticated PhD chemists in China, India and Pakistan and elsewhere can tweak the chemical constituents of "designer drugs" faster than law enforcement can even classify them as illegal.

Let's look at good old '60s **LSD**. It was sold on tiny squares of blotting paper that were sucked on in the mouth. It has a half-century of documented user history. Its hallucinogenic properties are well understood. It causes users to have altered perceptions of time, and see inanimate objects as human. It creates a condition called "synethesis", wherein a user can *feel* colors and *see* sounds!

169

LSD stories were common of people jumping out of windows to their death. Often, mortal combat with imaginary demons was experienced. In general the overall experience with LSD was so negative that few partook frequently!

Anyone who has ever used or known someone who has used LSD *knows what to expect.* "Bad trips" can occur, and the psychological effect of these can actually last a lifetime. It didn't kill very many users, but it ruined many lives. It's street name is "**acid**". Not many use it today. The key is knowing what to expect.

Enter the new era of "designer drugs". A new product, "synthetic LSD" often simply sold on the street as "LSD", is a substance known as "NBOMe". Its street name is "**Smiles**" or "**En-bombs**".

The trouble is, **it isn't LSD.** Not even close. It is something *far* more powerful and toxic. It actually has the bizarre effect of causing users to stab themselves repeatedly! It leads to delirium, paranoia, violence, rapid heartbeat….and death. It is sold on blotter squares exactly as LSD was sold. If a Smiles user expects the *known* real-LSD effects they are in for a very rude and possibly fatal awakening.

The media loves to put the word "synthetic" in front of anything they want to vilify, regardless of whether the "synthetic" product has anything at all in common with the "real" product. Guilt by association works every time.

BEWARE "SYNTHETIC MARIJUANA"

An important marijuana industry negative we must overcome is the soaring popularity of so-called "synthetic-marijuana".

This is a very dangerous designer street-drug known as **"Spice"**, **"Moon Rocks"**, **"K2"**, or **"Skunk"**. It is giving "genuine" marijuana a far worse reputation than it has already. It is one more potential nail in the legalization coffin.

The implication is: "If the _fake_ stuff is bad, the _real_ stuff must also be bad or worse." This is the guilt by association perpetrated by the clueless or bought-off media, and readily believed by the equally clueless public.

The "logical" conclusion among the readership is, if the _synthetic_ marijuana can kill, surely the "real marijuana " must also kill! Not at all so. Spice is over **_one-hundred times_** more powerful than marijuana. A tiny dose can have a huge effect. Use often leads to psychosis, stroke, heart attack and irreversible kidney damage. This is a far cry from the harmless, pleasant, sleepy-high induced by marijuana.

The FACT is that the _media_ constantly refers to Spice as "_synthetic marijuana_" simply because it is often sold having a similar ground-up-plant-material _appearance._ There is absolutely **NO** CHEMICAL CONNECTION between the two substances. Chemically it is NOT "synthetic marijuana" any more than it is "synthetic pizza!"

Marijuana (call it weed, pot, ganja, grass, Maryjane or whatever) is a natural healing herbal plant with many thousands of years of well- documented medicinal benefits. Its complex chemistry is extremely well known. It is harmless, especially compared to alcohol and tobacco. **Spice, 'synthetic marijuana" kills.** Of course so does tobacco.

Spice is a synthetic chemical [1-pentyl-3-(1-napththoyl) indole] or some derivative of it whose effects are known to be **one-hundred times more powerful than marijuana or any of its constituents.**

171

Kids buy it. Kids smoke it. Kids die. There are over a thousand documented deaths in youths, and countless near deaths, from Spice use. Kids that experiment with real marijuana don't die from it. Further, numerous studies have debunked the common assertion that marijuana is a gateway-drug leading to cocaine or heroin addiction and worse.

The Spice basic chemical itself is shipped (often from China) to the United States as a white powder usually labeled "Plant Food" or "Fertilizer". Then it is dissolved by the cartels in a solvent such as alcohol, and added to *any* ground-up plant material. It can also be delivered, as with LSD, infused on blotter-paper. We've seen no studies of what happens if you actually were to feed it to a house plant!

Giant illicit laboratories, many of which are in China, are churning out thousands of pounds of this toxic poison. It's often marketed to kids as a "safer alternative to traditional marijuana." Spice is *extremely* dangerous. In fact, as a headline in *Time Magazine* put it: "**China, has become the new front in the global drug war**".

The Chinese drug makers can tweak the specific chemical ingredients in Spice so fast, and produce and ship them in such massive quantities, that federal drug enforcement simply can't keep up with the changes.

"Wholesalers" buy the "fertilizer" and turn it into liquids by dissolving it in acetone or alcohol. Then they use the liquid to soak plant matter,dry it, and package it up in attractive shiny metallic baggies. The baggies are labeled "plant food" so that your local box store can sell them. And they do. Of course printed on the bags is the phrase: "Not intended for human consumption". Apparently kids are not considered "human" by Chinese chemists.

172

In 2015, poison control centers received reports of over 4,000 serious reactions to "synthetic marijuana", according to the AAPC (American Association of Poison Control Centers.) In Tuscaloosa County, Alabama, where one person died and two dozen were hospitalized near-death after ingesting Spice at a party, police declared a public safety crisis.

In spite of the facts about Spice the media continues to refer to it as "synthetic marijuana". This has led to many unsuspecting youths to start using Spice expecting a known marijuana high, and subsequently dying. Thanks media.

The worst, and perhaps most popular teen street drug readily available today is "**Bath Salts**". It is named after the similar-looking bath-soak Epson Salts. Bath Salts are basically a synthetic combination of cocaine and amphetamines. Consumption results in dehydration, hyperthermia, muscle trauma and kidney failure...and quite often death.

The scariest thing is that Bath Salts are sold over the counter in many cleaver disguises, _well known_ to most teens. It might appear as "Mephedone Plant Food". It may appear as "Jewelry Cleaner". The packages will always carry the warning: "Not For Human Consumption". As with Spice, it is virtually impossible for the federal government to keep up with the vast array of mislabeled similar deadly products available.

Bath salts are chemically designed to mimic a stimulant called "cathinone". This naturally occurs in "khat", a plant native to the Arabian Peninsula and East Africa. Chewing the leaves of khat creates a mild stimulating effect. Bath Salts are _thousands of times_ more powerful than khat.

Bath Salts act by massively increasing kids dopamine levels, their reward/pleasure molecule. It raises levels to addictive and *extremely dangerous* heights. It is said that snorting one line of Bath Salts is the equivalent of snorting ten lines of cocaine! This can easily be fatal.

The scariest fact of all is not only the on-line internet availability, but the low price. A quick search will find Bath Salts on sale for $15.00 a bag! Unfortunately, Spice and Bath Salts are not the only inexpensive street drugs that are readily available to our kids and young adults. There are others.

"**Ecstasy**" is yet another popular street drug among teens and young adults. Known as "E" or "XTC", this product was actually sold as a legal appetite suppressant in the '70s! Ecstasy and its variants are the drugs of choice for "raves".

 A rave is a wide-open impromptu party. Ectsasy is known medically as an "empathogen". It breaks down shyness and insecurity and greatly enhances the experience of dancing to loud music and light shows. Apparently it helps shy guys get laid! It also leads to perceptual distortions and can damage not only brain cells but other organs as well. A study by Rutgers University concluded that dehydration, hyperthermia, kidney failure and heart failure were the most common and often deadly side effects of using Ecstasy.

"**Special K**", also known as "Vitamin K" (or just plain "K") is the chemical "ketamine". Small doses (it can be injected) such as 25mg can have a calming effect, and put the user in a meditative state or introspective mood that wears off in an hour or so. Up to 100mg has an anesthetic effect making the user tired and dizzy. As the dose is increased, as is unfortunately usually the case, there is loss of coordination, respiratory distress, paralysis, cardiac distress, coma…and too often death.

"DMT" (dimethyltryptamine) is yet another potent hallucinogenic street drug that can be snorted, injected, smoked or eaten. It is a US Schedule I drug, and quite deadly in overdose.

"Magic Mushrooms" or "psilocybin" were more popular in the '60s and '70s, but can still be purchased easily. They contain a triptomine alkaloid, and have an hallucinogenic effect on the user. They can be eaten, but are often consumed in a tea preparation, or baked into "magic muffins". As with LSD, bad trips are not uncommon. A recent small study in England indicated a possible medicinal use treating severe depression. Magic Mushrooms physical resemblance to the "Deadly Nightshade" mushroom, which can kill, make hunting for them in the woods a very risky proposition.

"Peyote Buttons" are not a common street drug. They do show up from time to time. Originally used by North Mexican Indian tribes in religious ceremonies, and later by Southwest Native Americans, consumption creates a trance-like state.

"Quaaludes": Made famous in the book and movie *The Wolf of Wall Street*, "ludes" are the only street drug with which I have any direct familiarity. My youngest son was quite fond of them! I can blame myself in a way, because before I learned the truth about the safety of marijuana I pleaded with both my young sons to NEVER SMOKE MARIJUANA! I was as brainwashed by the media as anyone else. I couldn't have given a crap less about "ludes".

Chemically "methaqualone", it is a central nervous system depressant that acts as a sedative and hypnotic. Apparently it is hard to die from its use as evidenced by that fact that Jordan Belfort and my son are both seemingly-healthy and bright fully-functional adults!

The following three street drugs are *really* ugly:

"Angel Dust ". Known as "PCP" or "Semyl", chemically it is "phencyclidine". It was developed in the '50s as a legal anesthetic, but discontinued because of dangerous side effects. This crap causes the most violent behavior imaginable. Fox news reported about a man on PCP who bit his son's eyeball out and ate it! One becomes invincible. The idea of charging head first through a brick wall seems perfectly doable. Many try; many die.

"Flakka". Also known as "gravel", is chemically "alpha-pyrrolidnopentiophenone". First appearing in 2015, it may be the single most deadly street drug of all. It has been responsible for many deaths in Florida and Australia, and is rapidly spreading across the United States. Emergency-room doctors refer to it a "The Devil's Drug". Apparently a $5.00 bag can turn a teen into a violent zombie!

"Superman". This deadly killer street drug has not yet become popular in the United States. It is a mixture of Ecstacy and methamphetamines. Earlier in 2016 five young adults died violently at the "Time Creep Music Festival" in Buenos Aires, Argentina. Dozens more were hospitalized near death. GOD help us when it arrives on our shores.

Of great importance, when *any* of the above drugs are combined with heroin, as is *commonly* done, the dangers are greatly magnified.

I know I have left out a few well-known drugs (opium comes to mind). The above list should give any concerned parent some incentive to encourage the government to make harmless herbal marijuana much more accessible through decriminalization and de-scheduling or re-scheduling. Anything that can cut down on kids' use of deadly designer street drugs should be a no-brainer.

It is worthy of note that "new" street drugs once made their way to Europe first, then to the United States. This gave American authorities at least *some* advanced warning.   Most recently designer drugs are hitting our streets first. This is not a good trend.

Reports indicate that over the past decade as many as **four-hundred** designer street drugs have appeared in Europe and the United States. ***Most of these have never even been tested on animals, much less on humans.*** There is growing evidence that the *contaminants* in some of these street drugs are at least as deadly as the drugs themselves.

The tiniest molecular tweak that makes a new designer drug "legal" can create a new drug with dramatically different psychoactive effects. It is impossible to predict how a drug structure modification will affect potency, activity, or toxicology. The Chinese PhDs couldn't care less. Drug laws can't keep up with chemistry. The number of small molecular changes that can be made to any substance is almost infinite.

Our drug enforcement officials classify all designer street drugs as "Novel Psychoactive Substances" (NPSs). At least the enemy has a government name, unlike "Islamic Terrorism". If marijuana were legalized the billions of dollars that could be saved can be focused on NPS **EDUCATION**.

Please answer honestly: Would you rather have your kid smoke tobacco, swig vodka, experiment with the above deadly street drugs, or smoke a marijuana joint? Of course you would rather not have them do *any* one of these. Please ask yourself, looking realistically at the statistics, which one stands out as basically harmless, and by far the best choice? **MARIJUANA**! It is a no-brainer best choice.

Sadly, there are many who are totally convinced, after being subjected to a lifetime of lies and anti-marijuana propaganda, that marijuana is a gateway drug to the above far worse and more addictive street-drug substances. This has been proven to be false in many scientific studies.

To those uninformed individuals I ask: "Would you not rather have your kids or teens chill out on marijuana, which will make them *very* sleepy at worst and cannot possibly kill them, OR would you rather have them experiment with commonly-available street drugs **as they do today and will continue to do in the future, and very possibly die**?

No one today can reasonably argue that marijuana led their sons and daughters to these dangerous street drugs. Countless studies have determined that most street drug users never touched marijuana in the first place.

When I was a kid in the 1940s, many of the guys I knew sniffed model-airplane glue from a brown bag. It has been conclusively shown that medically this practice kills brain cells. Apparently sniffing alkyd-based paints worked equally well. This was before the era of non-sniffable water-based paints.

I can recall friends literally passing out, falling down, and injuring themselves in the process. I tried it once. It gave me a headache! I guess I lost a few brain cells in the process. Even today it is the cheapest "high" any kid can get. And many try it. This is the easiest "gateway drug" of all.

Of course alcohol is always readily available. Most kids find the "high" too unexciting and the resulting hangover too annoying. Yet a few do become lifelong alcoholics. Eventually some, like my mom, die from liver cirrhosis. Others, like my mom's mom, live forever!

Today there are the readily available street drugs described above that virtually **every kid tries at least once.** Studies have indicated that in *any given year* one in four kids, teens and young adults experiment with a deadly street drug. Some surveys show that the rate of use is much higher.

Some of these street drugs are **almost *instantly* addictive**. Some can kill rapidly. They are cheap, easy to use, and offer a variety of out-of-body experiences, many quite unpleasant, many deadly. In addition to the above designer street drugs are the "old standbys", **Crack Cocaine** , **Heroin,** and **prescription opiates.**

"Crack" is a white powder derived from cocaine. It is generally inhaled into the nose off some flat surface through a soda straw (known colloquially as "cutting a line"). Enough exposure turns the user into a toothless, wide-eyed stammering freak. I've met a few.

"Heroin", known on the street as "Horse" or simply "H", is deadly. It killed hilarious comedian John Belushi. It killed singer Janis Joplin. It killed Chris Farley and Mitch Hedburg and Lenny Bruce. It is highly addictive, commonly administered by injection. Use leads to heart attacks and strokes. It carries the double whammy of its users often falling victim to HIV from contaminated injection needles.

Prescription Opioids: Of course every mom and dad has an accessible bottle in a drawer or cabinet somewhere. Morphine, dilaudid, oxycontin....all powerful and deadly,

179

highly addictive pain killers. And kid killers. Prescription opioids recently killed the world-famous entertainer Prince.

Drug policies in countries such as the United States and England were drawn up long before the internet happened. The newly interconnected illicit drug scene has grown incredibly complex. Existing laws cannot be revised as fast as new designer drugs appear.

In just the last decade, the global trade in drugs has shifted in unpredictable and profound ways. The reality of designer street drugs in the digital age is that, on deep and complex web markets, as any kid knows <u>any illegal drug is just a click or two away</u>.

If you want to help and participate in our cause, please go to our informative website and sign up for our free newsletter. If you wish to support our cause in any way possible you can donate any amount on our extremely secure encrypted website at: TNWLF.org_ (The National Weed Legalization Fund).

Thanks!

CHAPTER 24
THE KILLER PRESCRIPTION DRUGS
WE ALL TAKE

Roger Pertwee, Chair of Neuropharmacology at the University of Aberdeen:
"At the moment, marijuana is in the hands of criminals, and that's crazy. Persons buying marijuana *illicitly* have no idea what the composition is, what has been added to it."

We have a serious **epidemic** in the United States today. It can be blamed directly on the drug manufacturers (Big Pharma), Big Tobacco, and Big Alcohol, aided by a complicit, tax hungry federal government. It is one of America's greatest shames.

In the preceding Chapter 23 I focused on "street drugs" as they relate to kids, teens and young adults. That was not to say that older adults do not use street drugs. It is just that most older individuals are beyond the "experimental stage", and, frankly, simply know better.

Sadly, they do not know better than to smoke, drink in excess, and take prescription painkillers!

The **deadliest** substances in America today are all **100% legal**!

1. Tobacco: Linked to 1 in 5 American **deaths**, **20%**!

2. Alcohol: Alcohol induced aggression is the major cause of domestic violence. Alcohol is implicated in **40%** of all violent crimes. Liver cirrhosis claims 26,000

lives a year, exceeded only by drunk driving which claims 62,000 lives.

3. Prescription opioid painkillers and other prescription drugs cause thousands of **deaths** every year.

DEATH? Do you even want to *consider* a pill that can kill you? Most already do. In fact, we all take them.

We do it so frequently we don't give it a second thought. The next time you pick up any prescription at your local pharmacy take the time to read the "instruction sheet" that accompanies it. You might also want to check the manufacturer's complete blurb pertaining to that drug, which is readily accessible on line. What you are looking for are the "contra-indications"

Most contra-indications are relatively mild. Upset stomach or a rash are pretty common. What I find disquieting is the frequency that the word "<u>death</u>" can almost always be found buried in the contra-indication fine print. I'm convinced the printing industry invented a special tiny print font intended just for prescription drug warnings that are nearly impossible to read without a magnifying glass!

Below is a very short list of a few drugs chosen at random for which I found multi-page ads in some of the magazines I read. I don't mean to pick on these particular drugs. I imagine they mention death to cover their legal asses "just in case" no matter how unlikely. I still find it scary.

- Xarelto. A drug intended for multiple sclerosis. There are many lawsuits outstanding. Apparently it can kill. I prefer my MS.

- Breo. Recent frequent TV commercials tout this asthma medicine. The announcer casually mentions "the possibility of death" in mid-commercial! Of course it is always "In Rare Cases" or "Rarely Noted", or "Seldom Seen" but it is still within the realm of the possible. I hate the possible!

- Nulasta . This cancer drug's instructions contain the words "fatal", and "death".

- Xifaxin. Intended to mitigate diarrhea, it points out a "possible fatal dose". Clog up with caution!

- OID. Stands for "opioid induced constipation". First they give you an addictive opioid, then they sell you an antidote for one of its less pleasant side effects! Marketing 101. Good job, Big Pharma!

- Xeljanz. Intended for rheumatoid arthritis, it is clearly stated that: "Some people have **died**..."! At least they no longer have pain.

- Pradaxa. Intended for blood clots: "Pradaxa can cause bleeding which can be serious and sometimes lead to **death**." Cool!

- Entresto: Intended for heart patients, it: "May cause angioedema that may cause trouble breathing and **death**." So much for the heart!

With a bit of research I could list hundreds. The sad fact is that these prescription drugs are all _perfectly legal_! Big Pharma has convinced (however they may have accomplished that) our federal government that these potential killers have a _greater upside than downside._ Of course, I cannot think of a worse downside than **death**. Can you?

That brings us to the single greatest drug tragedy facing America today, **prescription opioids.** These include oxycontin, oxycodone, Percoset, morphine, fentanyl, and dilaudid. I'm sure many of my readers are familiar with these frequently-prescribed pain killers. You have probably taken one or more in the past. I certainly have.

My Hawaii real estate partner Mike, a very intelligent and savvy guy, learned the about oxycontin the hard way. He injured his back on a construction job about ten years ago. He was prescribed oxycontin for pain relief. Over the next eight years he became *totally addicted*. He managed to total six cars. He was almost killed in one of the accidents.

As it is with most opioid addicts, he managed to find an army of doctors and a variety of pharmacies in more than one state at the same time. All would gladly supply him with an endless supply of "oxy". I seem to recall that radio commentator Rush Limbaugh had a similar experience a few years ago.

Mike spent eight years in and out rehabilitation. He lost his marriage. He lost his beautiful home. He lost all of his friends. In fact, he lost everything. It is a miracle he didn't lose his life. Today he is slowly coming out of his addiction, but it is a very long and painful road.

Oxycontin has been proven to be a gateway drug to heroin for many users. It is reported that heroin deaths have increased 40% over the past five years mostly due to oxycontin legal prescriptions. Big Pharma makes millions while consumers turn into addicts, criminals and corpses.

The statistics (also presented in Chapter 6) are astounding:

A study done in 2015 that was published in *The Annual Review of Public Health* showed some amazing numbers:

- Total sales of 72 kilograms (158 pounds) of pain killers per 100,000 people (a mere <u>276 tons</u>; that's a hell of a lot of little white pills);

- Deaths from overdoses were an astounding 54 per 100,000 people (over 189,000 individuals, an average of 500+ per day);

- Hospital admissions for overdoses was an amazing 410 per 100,000 people (over a million and a quarter (1,435,000) individuals! This is an average of more than 3,900 overdoses daily.)

This qualifies as a massive **AMERICAN EPEDEMIC**!

I am an Army veteran, and a member of American Legion Post #66 in Green Valley, Arizona. I am not afflicted with Post Traumatic Stress Disorder (PTSD). My next door neighbor Mike (a different Mike), a Vietnam veteran is, severely. So are many of the vets I speak with at the American Legion.

They all seek help at the Tucson Veterans Administration hospital. They are all hooked on opioids as well as anti-depressants. These are the only medicines the VA has until recently been able to legally offer them for relief. Big Pharma must literally make billions of dollars yearly on the backs of our brave veterans. It need not be so. It may change soon.

Now let's compare the above mentioned legal medications with a harmless herbal medicine in use *for thousands of years to mitigate pain.* It is called **MARIJUANA**! It has NEVER KILLED ANYONE. It cannot kill anyone.

Yet for some unfathomable reason our government, apparently in conspiracy with Big Pharma, keeps marijuana as a criminally illegal substance in the same Schedule I as crack cocaine and heroin. Truly amazing.

Our government is famous for some really bizarre stuff. Millions of taxpayer dollars have been spent on such nonsense as studying the sex life of goldfish and the treadmill efficiency of shrimp. The legendary $700 hammers and $400 toilet seats also come to mind. Or was it $700 toilet seats and $400 hammers? Whichever!

The totally useless new zillion dollar replacement Air Force fighter jet (it simply does not work!) for the incredible A10 aircraft is our latest expensive buffoonery. Billions more down the crapper. We never learn.

But failing to realize the value of marijuana as a medicine and as a harmless recreational pleasure, in spite of countless scientific studies and anecdotal evidence to the contrary, trumps them all!

I have yet to find *anyone* who can possible explain to me the logic behind this disgraceful on-going tragedy.

Not one.

CHAPTER 25
DID JESUS USE MARIJUANA?

Paul Hansen, Senior Pastor of Holy Spirit Lutheran Church in Las Vegas:
"On its face, our current marijuana laws appear to be moral, but it is a cosmetic morality. Our current laws are causing virtually unfettered access to marijuana. Marijuana is far easier to access than alcohol because drug dealers don't card."

Sometime many decades ago (the '60s) I believed that I had a calling to serve Jesus Christ. I studied diligently, and eventually became ordained and licensed as a Christian minister. Although to this day I do bereavement counseling, and an occasional friend's wedding, I decided after a few years that there were many other ways to serve GOD.

Once I became deeply involved in the marijuana legalization movement I wondered whether there was any biblical evidence of marijuana use, and whether the possibility existed that Jesus himself could have been a user.

Many great writers, painters and thinkers over the centuries are known to have gotten their inspiration and clarity of thought from smoking marijuana. Why not Jesus?

Many extremely religious individuals are totally against all drugs, including marijuana, on religious principal alone. It is one reason that very few politicians would ever advocate for legalization, regardless of their personal feelings on the matter. They fear the loss of this huge voting bloc. (They also fear the loss of whatever "perks" or campaign donations are being given to them by Big Pharma, but that's another story.)

So, do *you* think Jesus could possibly have been familiar with marijuana? A possible user? The fact is, no one knows! Nor could anyone possibly know, with the limited information about Jesus that we have at present.

Regarding early Judaism and Christianity I have read everything I can get my hands on written by Dr. Bart D. Ehrman, Professor, Department of Religious Studies, The University of North Carolina at Chapel Hill.

One thing Dr. Ehrman points out is that, for many decades after his death on the cross, nothing to date has ever been found that was written about the man called Jesus. There are no *contemporaneous* accounts of his life or his habits during this time period. Not one word. In fact, during the times shortly after Jesus' death he was not even considered an important figure, certainly not one worthy of documentation. Thus, this lack of historical data is not surprising.

Jesus may or may not have been literate. Thoughts vary on this. Only a single reported incident of him writing a short phrase in the sand with a stick indicates any degree of literacy. It is somewhat likely he could read but not write. But if he was literate and actually did keep a diary or journal no trace or reference has ever been found.

Almost nothing is known about Jesus' days as a child and as a youth. The recent movie is pure fantasy. It isn't even a certainty whether or not he was ever married in *later* life!

The Holy Bible as we know it today is a compilation of hundreds of years of translation, re-translation, scribes errors and personal insertions. It includes the often arbitrary decisions by various rulers as to what would become canon (fixed written laws) and what would not be included in the many "latest" versions. It is a "living document".

This is diametrically opposed in content to the Koran which is a fixed and unchangeable word for word book as set down by Mohammad himself as absolute canon. There can be no "modern translation" or "updated version" of the Koran. No Martin Luther cognate can exist. It is a "static document."

This in a sense is probably preferable to a Holy Book that has changed considerably over the centuries at the whim of various "authorities", and that has many "Book Ofs" that never even made it as canon into THE Book.

Studies conducted at the Hebrew University in Jerusalem have concluded that the word "cannabis" is actually derived from the Arabic "kunnab" which came from the Syric "qunnappa". This traces back still further to the Hebrew word "pannag". They claim that the Exekiel (27:17) reference to "pannag" is referring to cannabis.

There is also a school of thought that "kan bosm" = "Reed of Balm", referred to in the Bible, when translated into modern Hebrew is either "kannabos" or "kannabus".

Because marijuana use is clearly documented in China millennia before the life of Christ, it is certainly not inconceivable that marijuana was in common use throughout the Holy Lands in Jesus' times. This is especially true if one concedes that cannabis is in fact specifically mentioned in the Bible.

Saint John The Devine describes a tree whose leaves "were for the healing of the nations". Marijuana?

Would Jesus, a homeless, travelling Holy Man, with no obvious means of support, not today be considered a "hippie" of sorts? Hippies are traditionally thought of as chilled-out marijuana smokers.

Knowing the extent that marijuana is known to enhance the creativity among history's great thinkers, authors and painters, is it too great a stretch to believe that Jesus, a great philosopher and lecturer, also used marijuana in some form? Could his creative genius not only be Divinely inspired by The Father, but also enhanced by a harmless common medicinal herb?

Why is all of this of any importance? Well, if it were well documented that Jesus used marijuana, would it still be considered illegal in America today? Interesting conjecture.

I leave this matter open for the reader to ponder and decide. In my opinion, probability aside, Jesus use of "pannag" is certainly within the realm of the possible.

CHAPTER 26
STONED RABBITS

<u>Redman</u>, **Rapper/Musician:**
"Big up to Colorado and Washington for being the first states to pass marijuana legalization. They're not afraid."

The anti-marijuana crowd is *really* starting to scrape the bottom of the anti-legalization idea barrel!

It was reported in *The Daily Beast* that during hearings in Utah, Drug Enforcement Agent Matt Fairbanks made the argument that **IF** growing marijuana outdoors was, Heaven help us, *legalized* in Utah, that <u>the state's ecosystems would be in serious danger</u>.

Why, one might logically ask? Because Utah's storied, valued rabbit herds might nibble on the marijuana crop and get stoned. **You *can't* make this stuff up!**

I can see clearly now where this is all headed. Anyone, anywhere, desiring to grow marijuana is going to be required to provide an "<u>EIS</u>". This is the dreaded "Environmental Impact Statement" required by The Environmental Protection Agency. It is the bane of all real estate developers. Involving the <u>EPA</u> to muddy the waters and delay marijuana growing eternally would be a stroke of genius!

Can any potential marijuana grower in Utah (or anywhere else) unequivocally guarantee in an EIS that there will be no herd of raging maniacally stoned bunnies on the loose destroying everything in sight? Bye bye ecosystem?

For example, in my state of Arizona we have rules that strictly limit desert real estate development in the mythical "Spotted

Owl Habitat". Here's the rub: We are dealing with **_hypothetical_ habitat**. There are prohibited building areas where _no spotted owl has ever pooped, been seen, heard or documented!_

The argument is that _should,_ GOD forbid, a confused, off course, perhaps handicapped or sick, spotted owl someday actually accidentally fly over the area it might like it and decide to, gasp, _land_ there.....or even worse, _nest_ there, all hell would break loose! Heaven help us should we prevent it from doing so. Goodbye ecosystem. Why not the same argument for a future marijuana or hemp crop? Very scary.

So, you anti-marijuana folk, why not set about proposing legislation everywhere that declares **all** land "forever marijuana free". Base this on the argument that in the event some animal (rabbit, mouse, chicken, elephant, unicorn....whichever) should someday chomp on some marijuana and get stoned, the ecosystem would be destroyed for all eternity!

Bunny eats marijuana and gets stoned. A sleepy bunny is an easy kill for a hungry coyote. Chomp. Oops...coyote now fed, happy, and stoned. Takes a nap, gets eaten by a puma. Happy puma passes out on the road. Puma gets run over by an eighteen-wheeler. Ecosystem destroyed. Whatever.

You can't make this stuff up. The hysteria among the anti-marijuana crowd and their desperation in continuing to fight a losing battle against legalization is one of the most incredible social spectacles in America today. We can only pray that sanity prevails. Sadly it seldom does.

As an afterthought, the above nonsense just suggested a

great idea for Australia to adopt. Maybe their **pro**-marijuana-growing folks will catch on to this. It is based on the fact that Australia has far more rabbits than people, and they are considered a major pest to be eradicated at any cost.

I can vividly recall driving from Alice Springs to Uluru (Ayers Rock) one evening and seeing in my headlights the wind blow waves of leaves across the highway ahead of me, for mile after mile after mile. No, hold on, those aren't leaves...they're freaking rabbits! There had to have been " billions and billions" of them (sorry Carl)! They must thrive on red dirt because that is about the only thing I saw along that route that they could live on!

So here's my proposal, Australia. Plant marijuana everywhere. The rabbits will all eat it and get stoned out of their minds, collapsing in place in sheer ecstasy. Then, instead of expensive fencing, trapping, poisoning and hunting the ravenous little fur balls you simply scoop them up in front-end D10 bucket loaders and deposit them in garbage dump trucks! It's actually relatively humane. They'll never know the difference, and at least they'll all die happy!

I know, I know, nothing green grows in the outback. But ridding the sub-continent of the scourge of the ravenous little funny bunny by marijuana-stoning and mass-scooping the little critters is at least an entertaining idea!

With desperation setting in, can legalization be far behind!

CHAPTER 27
TESTING MARIJUANA, & DUIs

Chris Rock, **Actor and Comedian:**
"I'm all for the legalization of weed."

Marijuana plants are like snowflakes. No two are exactly alike. People are like snowflakes. No two individuals, not even identical twins, are *exactly* alike.

Hi! I'm Joe Fastfeet, a college football star and a top draft pick potential NFL player. I just got offered a multi-million dollar multi-year contract. I gladly submitted to a drug test. Why not? I don't do drugs.

Ooops! *I just learned that failed my drug test and lost my contract.* How the hell did that happen? Must be some mistake! **I don't *do* drugs**.

Uh, Hi Joe! Remember me? Remember that college dorm party we were at a month or so ago? We were all pretty damn drunk! Remember I passed you a joint? You didn't want it, but you took a drag just to make me happy! You coughed your fool head off! We all wet ourselves laughing! Remember that, Joe?

Case in point: Marijuana is fat soluble, and traces of it, even after ingesting a small amount, can be detected in your system *weeks later*! You're screwed Joe. You're an official stoner. No amount of explaining can ever change that test result. No one will ever believe you don't use marijuana regularly. Have fun flipping burgers!

Could this really happen? Yes, it could. It depends on a

number of different factors:

- How much THC was in that strain you smoked?
- How much CBD was in that strain you smoked?
- How long did you keep the smoke in your lungs?
- How much second hand marijuana smoke was in the room while you were present?
- How long were *you* in the room?
- How much do you weigh?
- Do you know the infinite details of your personal physiology?

It's unlikely Joe could honestly answer most of these questions. Joe was at that dorm party and tested positive weeks later. Another person present might have tested negative. Everyone is affected differently by marijuana.

Until you try marijuana and experiment with it, working with different strains and different doses, no one, no doctor, no dispensary owner, can give you a certain idea of what effect you can expect *or* how long it remains testable in your body.

Body weight and body fat percentage are one factor, but there are dozens of other personal physiological factors that come into play as well. No one could possibly predict how long after using any given amount of marijuana you might still test positive.

This is why police DUI testing for marijuana is at best futile, at worst almost criminal. What might impair one driver to the extent that he is a danger to anyone within fifty miles, might have absolutely zero impairment effect on a different driver.

Some states recognize this and will only arrest and convict on a DUI if the driver is in actual physical possession of marijuana. Some states will conduct on-site impairment tests such as walking a straight line.

I can tell you from personal experience as a balance-challenged multiple sclerosis patient that there is no way I can walk a dead-straight line! I'll get busted for impairment any time I get pulled over and that particular test is conducted. (P.S. I have not had even a minor car accident in forty years or more and I drive over 50,000 miles a year.)

Unfortunately some other states will be conducting *blood and urine* marijuana DUI tests, often on the spot. Unlike alcohol impairment, which diminishes rather quickly with time, such is not the case with marijuana. These will be the problem states for medical and recreational marijuana users who drive.

If I smoke a strong joint today, the actual effect of which wears off after about four hours, and I get pulled over, I'll be busted via a blood test for anywhere from three to six weeks from today This is in spite of the fact that my driving impairment has been ZERO for all of those entire three to six weeks!

In fact, there are absolutely no studies that I can find that indicate any particular amount of marijuana detected can be reconciled with any given individual's level of impairment. The marijuana-specialty attorneys should have a field day with this one. They already advertise this specialty!

There is on the internet lots of ready advice on how to beat a marijuana DUI. One way is the use of concealed urine receptacles that can be worn under clothes and pre-filled with clean piss! I'll leave it up to my readers to check these out themselves!

Every state will require careful, accurate testing of all marijuana intended for medical use. Marijuana intended for recreational use may not be as strictly tested. They will certainly require tests for contaminates such as pesticides and mold, and approximate THC and CBD levels.

Home test kits have been developed that enable anyone to do a rough analysis of the major components in a sample of marijuana. They are relatively inexpensive, but certainly do not produce the accurate analyses available from a serious laboratory. Someday some genius will invent a really accurate and simple home test, patent it, and make a fortune!

The available home test is based on a process known as "chromatography". There are three basic types, liquid, thin-layer, and gas. For anyone interested in the minute details of these home analytical methods I suggest the excellent short book *Cannabinoids and Terpenes* published by Ryder Management.

Setting up a state-approved laboratory is a very expensive proposition. It can run into hundreds of thousands of dollars. From a staffing standpoint, the head honcho is usually a PhD organic chemist. There may also be a physician involved. Operators of the technical scientific equipment involved are highly skilled and well paid, and may have a chemistry or engineering background as well.

Because of the complexity of marijuana, accurate testing is not easy. Scientists have identified over four-hundred component compounds! The most important of these are THC and CBD and their many variants, as well as the many critical terpenes and flavonoids.

Chromatography is employed in many analytical labs, but it has accuracy limitations. The primary analytical equipment employed today is called a "mass spectrometer". The analyses provided by the medical dispensary that I frequent lists around twenty marijuana component percentages down to two decimal places (e.g. THC = 17.68%), accuracy that only a mass spectrometer can achieve..

Wikipedia (wikipedia.org) defines the mass spectrometer process as: "An analytical technique that ionizes chemical species and sorts the ions based on their mass to charge ratio. In simpler terms, a mass spectrum measures the masses within a sample. Mass spectrometry is used in many different fields and is applied to pure samples as well as complex mixtures." Right on.

From the standpoint of future marijuana industry employment, any college-age teen might well consider chemistry, particularly organic chemistry, as a road to follow. Combining that degree with a knowledge of marijuana that can be learned from books and the internet (see Appendix II) should position him or her very well to obtain high-paying employment as the marijuana industry expands nationwide.

At this time every state must have its own in-state analytical laboratories. In Hawaii each *Island* must have one. It is illegal to mail or ship marijuana samples inter-state or iner-Island for test purposes.

All such restrictions should change in a decade or so as America becomes more enlightened about **Marijuana – The Wonder Weed!**

CHAPTER 28
"DRY LAB" & A PARADOX

AN INCONVENIENT TRUTH

Snoop Dogg, Rapper:
"If marijuana were legal, there would be less high-speed chases, less robberies, less crime. Go to Amsterdam or The Netherlands where it is legal and you see that the crime rate is nonexistent. There are people riding on bicycles being happy and it's because of the environment that's provided by the legalization of marijuana. Alcohol was legalized so it could be taxed. If you legalize marijuana, it'll save lives and will put more money in the financial side, so why not?"

What I am about to offer in this Chapter might come as a shock to many. It will be refuted. It is, however, written based on my personal experience. From many peer discussions I know for a fact I am not alone in my knowledge of this matter.

I graduated from the Brooklyn Polytechnic Institute with a Bachelor's Degree in Chemical Engineering. At the time BPI was universally rated as one of the three top engineering schools in the country, along with MIT and CalTech. (It is now known as NYU Poly, and sadly much less highly regarded.)

Among my professors were top names in engineering circles worldwide such as Dr. Timochenko and Dr. Donald Othmer. Their college texts are still in use to this day. My point is I know more than a thing or two about lab work. Many of my friends are far more sophisticated "lab rats" than I, such as my best childhood friend who earned his PhD in organic chemistry, a far more lab-intensive discipline then ChemE. They all confirm what I relate below.

The term "**DRY LAB**" refers to the immoral practice of creating a best case scenario out of worst case data! This practice is one of making up lab results that perhaps never happened and publishing misleading conclusions based on these fantasy results.

In the *worst* case Dry Lab scenario, if one's lab results were skewed in favor of a result for which you were neither hoping nor expecting, you simply switch the samples! Voila! Another successful experiment!

Was this a *common* practice in my college lab? Probably not, but it definitely *did* occur. If someone got a particularly outstanding result of an experiment we'd tease: "Dry labed it again?" Who knew?

At one point in my eclectic corporate career I was Director of Special Projects for a Division of a Fortune 500 company. Their focus was primarily on various chemicals used in fossil fueled and nuclear power generating plants.

On one field trip I was monitoring the use of a proprietary chemical designed to prevent corrosion in the long thin copper tubes conducting cooling water. I was sad to find after analyzing my data that not only was our treatment ineffective, it actually *caused* some minor corrosion! Rats. My boss at that time was essentially an evil genius, a man of many talents but very few moral scruples.

When I reported my findings to him upon my return his response was: "Well Anderson, you know what to do, right?"

In my naiveté I said: "OK, we'll scrap this project and move on to test another product." My bad!

I was then subjected to a fifteen minute screaming lecture on Corporate responsibility to stockholders, Corporate credibility, Corporate greed, and the "Prime Directive". "General Order #1": NEVER admit failure, even in the face of overwhelming evidence to the contrary.

His orders: "Damn it, Anderson. Just publish the results but switch the samples so it looks like we actually prevented corrosion rather than caused it". That was a classic real-world example of "Dry Lab"!

I probably should have quit on the spot, but I had a fabulous high-paying job with unlimited worldwide travel and an unlimited expense account, so personal greed won the day and I said: "Yes Sir." But I then proceeded to go about my business as usual, shit-canned the report, and never heard another word about it!

What is my point in relating this story? Simply that I do not fully believe ANY marijuana test results that are published, regardless of who conducted the study or what conclusion was "proven". This pertains to studies that prove the effectiveness and safety of marijuana, as well as to those that confirm that it is, indeed, "The Devil's Lettuce".

I am not suggesting that the doctors or whomever is in charge of studies are always complicit. It is surely within the realm of possibility that the lab rats doing the actual testing-lab scut-work might Dry Lab a result here and there for the sake of expedience.

This is why I consider anecdotal evidence, the sworn reports of actual users, to have far more validity than any

published lab reports will *ever* have.

Am I alone in this conclusion? Apparently not.   An editor of the prestigious *New England Journal of Medicine* Dr. Marcia Angell is quoted as saying:

"It's simply no longer possible to believe much of the clinical research that is published, or rely on the judgment of trusted physicians or authoritative medical guidelines. I take no pleasure in this conclusion which I reached slowly and reluctantly over my two decades as editor."

One other point I'd like to mention. During the countless lectures and courses on mathematics and probability theory to which my young mind was painfully subjected I recall learning something called "Simpson's Paradox".

Wikipedia definition: "Simpson's paradox, or the Yule– Simpson effect, is a paradox in probability and statistics, in which a trend appears in different groups of data but disappears or ***reverses*** when these groups of data are combined. It is sometimes given the impersonal title of reversal paradox or amalgamation paradox."

It has been proven that when conducting any laboratory test where there are various sets of data (which is true in almost *every* long-term medical marijuana test) that if one combines the sets of data into one set and draws conclusions from it, one may get the **exact opposite** result s than if one considers the separate data as standalones.

I wonder how many of the marijuana studies being done today take Simpson's paradox into consideration? How many lab Directors consciously decide not to?   Could someone not selectively decide whether or not to consider applying it just to prove their personal viewpoint?

Any guesses?

CHAPTER 29
"LEGAL" MARIJUANA AND YOUR LIVELIHOOD

Neal Boortz, **Syndicated Radio Host & Author:**
"I'm for drug legalization. That doesn't mean that I'm for drug abuse... I'm convinced that we can do a better job...at a lower price...of handling our drug problem in this country through treatment rather than through law enforcement."

OK, so you live in a state where marijuana is legal for medicinal purposes. You have a serious medical condition, such as multiple sclerosis, and have found that marijuana helps you maintain a normal life. You find a delivery system that works for you, smoking, vaping, sub-lingual tinctures or yummy brownies! And you partake daily.

Or perhaps you live in one of the five places where recreational use is legal, and you find that instead of a martini after dinner a bit of marijuana is far more pleasing and far less harmful.

As with most folks not on permanent welfare, you actually *work* for a living. You hope to continue to do so. You are good at your job, punctual, accurate, and considered a very valuable employee. Your family depends on that paycheck.

Oops! Unlucky you. You work for one of the *many* American companies that have a zero-tolerance drug policy, including marijuana. And double oops, they just did a random drug test on you. Surprise! They found marijuana in your system, a total no-no. You have a pink slip in your future.

Of course you explained to Human Resources that the medical marijuana in your system is what makes you the valuable employee that you are. And they fired you that very same day. Illegal? Unconstitutional? Not at all!

Remember when your mom or dad used to tell you, in response to one of your rebellious teenage acts, that it was "their house, their rules"? Unfortunately marijuana legalization issues are creating similar reactions from employers. "Their company, their rules." These actions are aimed directly at employees who are ignoring the company policy of zero drug tolerance.

It matters not one bit that marijuana has been legalized in your state. It matters not one bit that you cannot function without your medical marijuana. You are exhibiting criminal company behavior! End of story.

Unrealistic scenario? Just ask Eugene, Oregon television news anchor Cyd Maurer. The AP reported that she was fired from her job at her zero-tolerance network for testing positive for marijuana. It was perfectly legal for them to fire her. Written Company Policy. No exceptions. Zero tolerance.

Of course Ms. Mauer could go home every night and drink an entire bottle of vodka and no one would give a damn. And if she was a smoker and used her cancer- sticks in an approved area at work that would be OK too. But to have a tiny residual amount of a harmless medicinal herb in her system detectable in a random blood test now THAT is simply unacceptable criminal behavior sufficient for termination.

After her firing, Ms. Maurer became a marijuana activist.

Check out her website at: askmeaboutmarijuana.com. The website points out the hypocrisy behind company policies that ban certain substances, like marijuana, but not others such as alcohol and tobacco. She shares her story in a video:

"I wasn't fired because I couldn't do my job. I wasn't fired because of my work ethic, my attitude, or my abilities. I was fired for enjoying a plant, on my own time, in the privacy of my own home. A plant that the majority of voters in Oregon believe should be legal." It IS legal in Oregon.

This is just one example of many similar scenarios played out nationwide. There is clearly a disconnect between company policy and legal employee behavior outside of work. You can and will be fired, quite legally, for using marijuana if it is against your company's "zero drugs" policy. It is irrelevant whether or not it is legal in your state.

The fact is that, because marijuana is still very unfortunately illegal federally, many companies are simply frightened out of their wits that in some way allowing their employees to use marijuana, whether or not it has any effect at all on their job performance, could somehow get them in deep doo doo with Uncle Sam. **The sad fact is that they could be right.**

One big problem for the marijuana user is that marijuana is detectable so long after its use. Smoking a single joint can lead to a positive test many weeks later! Being fat soluble it stays in your body far longer than traces of alcohol. It can be detected long after you are even remotely under its influence.

You can assume the risk and continue to use marijuana and risk failing a random drug test. You could just wait things out, and see if company policies change. The choice is yours, but keep in mind that simply because marijuana is legal in your state, your employer is still playing legal catch- up.

The moral of this story? If your company has a zero-tolerance drug policy you need to choose between being employed there, changing jobs to a more enlightened company, or staying put and not enjoying the many benefits of nature's Wonder-Weed, marijuana. Or you could simply risk continued use and hope you are never randomly tested.

Which would you choose?

CHAPTER 30
WANT TO START
A LEGAL DISPENSARY?

Woody Harrelson, Emmy Award-Winning Actor:
"I do smoke, but I don't go through all this trouble just because I want to make my drug of choice legal. It's about personal freedom. We should have the right in this country to do what we want, if we don't hurt anybody. Seventy-two million people in this country have smoked pot. Eighteen to twenty million in the last year. These people should not be treated as criminals."

Many entrepreneurs are hopping on the legal marijuana bandwagon. Selling this miracle medicinal herb out of licensed dispensaries sounds like the road to riches. It isn't. Yet. Perhaps never.

Anyone who has ever actually run any sort of brick-and-mortar business knows that the ONLY reason they can make *any* money is the complex but business-friendly United States Internal Revenue Service zillion-page Tax Code.

I recently spoke with the owner of a local dispensary. After only a few months in business he is seeking a buyer after his first visit to his CPA! When he started the business he figured that he could sell marijuana for at least twice what he was paying for it wholesale. It seemed to be a no brainer. Massive certain profit! Go for it.

He rented a nice store, renovated and furnished it, and hired staff to run it. He pays for heating and air conditioning, trash disposal, cleaning services, security, and all of the supplies needed to run his marijuana business in accordance with local codes and the complex state and federal laws.

Then reality set in. His CPA broke the news that he would be paying corporate taxes on his *GROSS* INCOME….every dime he took in. Why? Because the single biggest obstacles to starting any marijuana business where you "touch the plant" (as in a grow facility, dispensary, concentrator, laboratory, or edibles manufacturer) are the mind boggling and often confusing federal tax codes. The problem stems from the fact that marijuana is *federally illegal*, period.

Under federal law marijuana is a Schedule I controlled substance. He simply is not allowed under federal tax law to deduct his expenses and thereby pay taxes on only his NET INCOME, if any, *after* expenses, as with other businesses. Oops!

In 2015 the Ninth Circuit Court of Appeals upheld earlier rulings that preclude any marijuana business that "touches the plant" from the ability to claim most ordinary business expenses for tax purposes. This ruling echoed the earlier United States Tax Court rulings in upholding these absurd IRS restrictions.

These tax breaks are a common right afforded to *all* other American businesses. The simplest definition of "profit" is the revenue generated less the cost of generating it. Tax breaks are *the* key component.

To add insult to injury, there is an additional "Catch 22". Both state and federal taxing authorities automatically assess a **10% tax penalty** for not paying payroll taxes using electronic systems such as the EFTPS (Electronic Federal Tax Paying System). This is a penalty assessed on the *total tax burden*. Those businesses that touch the plant, however, are denied the *ability* to actually utilize the systems required to *prevent* the penalty from being assessed! **Catch 22.**

Well, it turns out that, at his tax rate, paying taxes based on his *gross* sales actually leaves him with a net loss! What a shocker. All of those expenses that would have reduced or perhaps even eliminated all of his taxes were now out of pocket. This is how huge multi-national corporations very often entirely legally manage to pay zero taxes. If they had to pay taxes on gross sales they'd ALL be out of business.

Let's look at an hypothetical example:

ANY ORDINARY BUSINESS:
Gross Receipts:	$2,000,000
Cost of Goods Sold	$ 900,000
Gross Profit	$1,100,000
Business Expense	$ 600,000 (tax deductible)
Net Taxable Income	$ 500,000
Tax @ 45% Rate	$ 225,000
Net Income	$ 275,000 (gross profit –
expenses - taxes)	

MARIJUANA BUSINESS "TOUCHING THE PLANT":
Gross Receipts:	$2,000,000
Cost of Goods Sold	$ 900,000
Gross Profit	$1,100,000
Business Expense	$ 600,000 (non-deductible)
Net Taxable Income	$1,100,000
Tax @ 45% Rate	$ 495,000
Net Income	$ 5,000! (= gross profit -
expenses - taxes)	

Add the "Catch 22" penalty, and you're out of business

fast! Perhaps this explains why I have seen a significant turnover of dispensary ownership here in my local Tucson area! In Marketing 101 finding a buyer for a failing business is called "The Greater Fool Theory".

Of course, Mr. Dispensary could simply raise his retail prices, no? Well, no! As it is now the black market illegal marijuana street vendors are having a ball. Because of the costs imposed by regulations associated with state and federal seed-to-sale tracking the price at which a dispensary must sell their products to make a profit, even if paying *net* taxes, is far higher than black-market street prices!

Legally-grown marijuana wholesale prices can exceed $2,000 a pound, and retail around double that, depending upon where you live. Illegal street-marijuana often sells for half of that! This disparity may be the long-term downfall of the entire legal marijuana industry.

The long-term solution is to eliminate the illegal drug trade. Lots of luck with that! After decades and billions of federal dollars the "War On Drugs" has been a dismal failure. I can go to virtually any city in the United States and in one hour I can find someone selling any and every street drug you can name, certainly including marijuana.

Here's another REAL problem for the potential dispensary owner. Let's look at Montana. There are dozens of operating dispensaries. The Montana Supreme Court has recently ruled that the entire medical marijuana program *must be eliminated* by August 2016! Every once-legal dispensary MUST shut down. The Montana Cannabis Industry Association has asked for delays and been granted some, but closures look inevitable.

Is this the absolute end of the medical marijuana movement in Montana? No, the public can still vote on a new program if one ever appears on the ballot. Will this Montana scenario give pause to ANY potential dispensary owner anywhere in the country in the future? Absolutely.

Need yet another reason to shy away from being a dispensary owner? Let's look at start-up costs. Every state is different. Some, those that clearly want to encourage the existence of dispensaries, keep the licensing fees reasonable. Other states, however, are determined to keep the little guy out. They only allow groups with very deep pockets to participate.

Hawaii is a perfect example of the latter. Earlier in 2016 they awarded eight licenses after receiving sixty-six applications. Applicants who won a license got shocked financially right away. They will have to pay **$75,000** to the state for their permit. The license winners then must pay **$50,000 annually** in renewal fees ! Ouch!

License winners must also show that they have $1 million in capital reserves plus $100,000 for each dispensary location granted. Could you come *close* to meeting these licensing costs? These costs MUST be passed on to the consumer. And as they are, cartel-supplied marijuana price spreads becomes wider and wider. The cartels are salivating!

There are many reasons why the federal government simply MUST un-classify or re-classify marijuana. Most often overlooked is the fact that keeping marijuana as a Schedule I drug makes it virtually **impossible** for any marijuana entrepreneur who "touches the plant" to make a living. **If any single factor in the long battle for legalization is critical to the success of the entire industry it is this onerous tax situation.**

211

CHAPTER 31
GROW ME IF YOU CAN – OR DARE!

<u>Michael Medved,</u> **Syndicated Radio Host:**
"We really should leave people alone to grow whatever plants they want. I don't want government to extend to supervising what people grow in the backyard. Do I believe that someone should go to jail because he is a midnight toker? No I don't. Most Americans would agree. Since we regulate prescription drugs, certainly regulating marijuana pretty carefully seems to me appropriate."

Marijuana is a weed. Weeds in general are rather hardy plants. Marijuana growing instructions in infinite detail are readily available on line and in many fine books. The plants are not particularly hard to grow.

The downside? **PRISON!** Growing marijuana yourself is illegal almost everywhere in the United States. Even in those twenty-six venues that have passed laws for medical and even recreational use, growing your own marijuana is severely restricted, if allowed at all.

For those who can *legally* grow marijuana, there are countless instructions available on the internet. There is also an excellent book: Ed Rosenthal's *Marijuana Growers Handbook* contains endless details within its 500+ pages on every conceivable aspect of cultivating marijuana. Another great book is *The Cannabis Grow Bible* by Greg Green.

The primary choices to be made by potential future legal growers are:

- Natural or synthetic fertilizers;
- Indoor or outdoor cultivation;

- Natural or artificial lighting;
- Grow in soil, in water (hydroponically), or in air (aeroponics);
- Temperature control and ventilation methods;
- Method of drying and processing;
- Security;
- Are you growing for high potency or high yield?
- What strains will you grow?
- Are you ready to pay a hundred dollars or more for ten seeds?
- How do the people you live with feel about this project?
- Do you have the time to tend to your plants?
- Do you have the patience to wait many months for your product?
- Are you prepared to shell out serious cash for growing equipment?
- Are you prepared for a MUCH higher electric bill?
- Are there any pets around who could damage your plants or cause a fire?
- Are there any kids around who could damage your plants or cause a fire?

Note that most dispensary licenses come with a grow license. It is strongly suggested that you **NEVER** grow marijuana unless you own a dispensary and/or have a medical marijuana card *and* you have written permission to grow on your property.

This does not stop thousands of exceptionally motivated risk takers from growing at least a few plants in every state and territory, authorities and their stupid laws be damned!

Some day in the far distant future growing may be legal, but for now it is 100% illegal both federally and in each individual state and territory, unless you have difficult-to-obtain permission.

If you decide the risk is worth it (it isn't), here are a few things to consider :

- How secure is your grow area?
- If indoors, how do you plan to hide the intense smell when the plants flower?
- Are *you* 100% tight lipped?
- Is EVERYONE in your house 100% tight lipped?
- Is there anyone you can trust to tend the plants in your absence?
- Are neighbors ever going to walk past your outside grow area and rat you out?
- Do you know what your legal rights are?
- Are you fully aware of your state's laws? Federal laws?
- Are you aware of the fines or jail time if you are caught?
- Are you aware that growing a single plant could carry similar penalties as for a larger grow?
- Can you afford a top attorney?
- Are you aware of the risk/reward ratio equation, i.e., $$$$ vis a vis jail time?
- Can your children be taken from you if you are caught and convicted?
- Will you lose your 9 to 5 job if you are caught and convicted?
- Are you aware you will never be employable in the marijuana industry in the future if you are caught and convicted?
- Can a legal gun or legal drugs present in your

home be used against you at trial?
- **Do you really *want* to risk this?**

Note that a grower can only influence a marijuana plant to reach a genetically inherent level of optimal growth to produce the largest quantity of THC that the particular plant is capable of producing. THC quantity is related to bud mass and how much resin can be collected from that bud mass.

Depending on the strain of a healthy outdoor marijuana plant will, it can produce between one and ten pounds of medicine. This is truly incredible because $2,000 - $3,000 a pound is not an unrealistic wholesale price. Does this mean a single huge plant could be worth $30,000? Yup! Do the math!

Back in the '70s black market Emerald Triangle (northern California) marijuana could fetch $8,000/pound!

In most states a dispensary license is accompanied by a license to grow specified quantities of marijuana. The profit potential is enormous. This is why cartels are planting *their* crops physically inside the crop plots of legal mass growers.

Especially in Colorado this has become a massive *new* problem in the generally futile War On Drugs. Only time will tell what effect this will have on the entire nationwide marijuana market and on the legalization movement itself.

MARIJUANA SEED BANKS

There are many companies dealing in marijuana seeds. Please check their websites for details. Seeds can cost at least $10.00 *each*, not exactly your $1.97 Burpee Seed marigold pack!

Archive Seed Bank   archiveseedbank.com

CBD Crew   cbdcrew.org (Europe)

Devil's Harvest	thedevilsharvestseeds.com
Elemental Seeds	elementalseeds.com
GrandDaddy Purp	granddaddypurp.com
Hortilab Seeds	hortilabseeds.com
Karma Genetics	karmagenetics.com
LaPlata Labs	laplatalabs.com
MTG Seeds	mtgseeds.com
Rare Dankness	raredankness.com
Reggae seeds	reggaeseeds.com (Spain)

Again, if you decide to grow your own marijuana, it is highly recommended that you ONLY do so if you have the *legal right* to do so. The federal government has its laws. Every state makes its own laws. **Obey them!**

Until that day in the far distant future when there will be universal recreational use and individuals can grow as much marijuana as they want, most legal marijuana horticulture in the USA will continue to be severely limited.

Live with it!

CHAPTER 32
CASH IN *NOW* –
GET A MARIJUANA JOB TODAY

Sarah Palin, **Ex Alaska Governor, VP Nominee:**
"We need to prioritize our law enforcement efforts, and if somebody's gonna smoke a joint in their house and not do anybody else any harm, then perhaps there are other things that our cops should be looking at to engage in and try to clean up some of the other problems that we have in society that are appropriate for law enforcement to do."

The opportunities for employment in the legal marijuana business are TREMENDOUS! As each new state either allows medical marijuana, or goes on to the next step, full recreational marijuana, the employment opportunities rapidly expand.

This is not to say you MUST reside in a state where marijuana is legal to find a good paying job in the industry. As you will see from the list below, there are many internet- based job possibilities that can be run from anywhere in your pajamas!

As with most decent paying jobs knowledge is king. Next in importance comes experience. If you have experience in a related niche that is a *big* plus. An example would be working at a bakery as an entree to making marijuana-laced cookies and brownies.

If you happen to be a marijuana user (preferably legal) and really know your products you will also have a leg up on a total newbie who has never used, regardless of the job you seek.

217

There are already literally thousands of jobs in the twenty or so states with operating dispensaries, grow facilities, edibles creators and testing laboratories. For the most part these positions are already filled, but there is always attrition. New jobs are available every day in these legal venues.

With diligent study you can become a very valuable expert in a field in which you may know absolutely nothing at the present time. There is almost infinite marijuana knowledge to be had by studying the internet and social media. Appendix II of this book lists many valuable internet resources you can access. It will take time, but study can change your life.

There are also well over a hundred excellent books available on every aspect of marijuana. Many of these can be found at your local library, or ordered from Amazon used or new. I've included a representative list of in Appendix II as well.

If you prefer structured education, check out Oaksterdam University (oaksterdamuniversity.com). They are considered in the industry to be a prime source of marijuana education.

There are also periodic, almost monthly, major marijuana business conferences across the country. Attendance is relatively expensive. By attending you will be exposed to hundreds of vendor exhibits and the opportunity to chat with vendors and attend educational seminars.

Two recent examples of these are the "Marijuana Business Conference and Exposition" held in Orlando, Florida May 9 – 11, 2016, and the cannabis "Business Summit and Exposition" June 20 – 22, 2016 in Oakland, California. You can easily find upcoming conferences with a Google search. You should definitely attend one or more. Learn, learn, learn!

You should also consider getting a subscribing to *High Times* magazine. It has been a standard marijuana publication for decades. In short, there is absolutely no reason why you cannot become a self-educated "expert" and have a serious employment advantage over almost everyone else seeking employment in this newly emerging market sector.

In Chapters 30 and 31 I go into some detail on owning a marijuana dispensary, and owning a grow facility. There is a great deal to learn about these two potential ventures. Both are very expensive to start, and can be difficult to run, and even difficult to show a profit, but for some it can be a road to marijuana riches.

But you do not have to actually OWN a dispensary or OWN a grow facility. There are a large number of good paying jobs created within these ventures. You could easily find yourself landing one of them if you take the time to learn the industry.

Let's take a hypothetical situation. Pennsylvania recently approved medical marijuana. It will probably be at least until late 2017 before they are ready to set up dispensaries and grow facilities. It is a large state with lots of potential medical users. There will be lots of new jobs available.

You have many months to learn as much as you can about marijuana before the new Pennsylvania laws are implemented. For example, you have lots of time to start working at a bakery while learning about marijuana.

How about starting work at a lab while gaining marijuana knowledge? You don't need a degree to start at the bottom in a lab running errands and cleaning glassware!

You have many months to learn any of the skills mentioned below. Do you not think you will have a *huge* advantage over the general job-seeking population if you can present a resume showing you have achieved skills that **very few** other applicants have? That you alone have knowledge in a specific area (such as baking) **AND** a thorough knowledge of marijuana? Finding a job should be a slam dunk!

If not Pennsylvania in 2017 or 2018 then where? There are the two dozen venues at present where medical marijuana is permitted. There are the five venues where full recreational use is allowed. More are expected to come on board later in 2016. Potential employment in this emerging industry is truly massive and even *now* available from coast to coast.

Keep in mind that there are two fundamental "types" of marijuana operations. There are those that "touch the plant" (growers, dispensaries, etc.) and those that "do not touch the plant" such as a head shop.

There is almost no business service that you can possibly imagine that the emerging legal marijuana industry does not need. Many of these are the common services that virtually all businesses need: legal, accounting, tax, etc. But many jobs that will be in great demand are *specific* to this budding industry. (Pun intended!)

The more states that come on board the more opportunities will exist. **The more marijuana knowledge you acquire the better positioned you will be to be hired!**

Here are some general areas of possible employment:

- Art
- Bakeries
- Building
- Candy Making
- Caregiving
- Creating Concentrates
- Domain Names

- Energy
- Events
- Greenhouses
- Home Delivery Services
- Horticulture
- Human resources
- Information & Training
- Laboratories
- Logo Creation
- Marketing
- Novelty Items
- Obtaining Grants
- Owning A Dispensary
- Owning a Head Shop
- Professional Services
- Raising Capital
- Real Estate
- Sales & Promotion
- Security
- Testing Labs
- Topicals & Lotions
- Website Creation

The following are some specifics of potentially available jobs:

PROFESSIONALS:

If you happen to be a professional, licensed as an attorney, doctor, accountant, real estate agent, securities broker or insurance agent you have an *amazing* opportunity to SPECIALIZE in marijuana matters. I have noticed a few attorneys in Arizona already advertising their expertise in the marijuana field.

The industry NEEDS professional help in each area.

Individuals who know the nuances and unique governing laws of a given venue, and can help navigate the complex web of regulations, will be well positioned for great paying jobs.

If you do not happen to possess a professional license, there are a number of very important college degrees one can obtain that relate directly to the marijuana industry.

A degree in agriculture could be especially valuable. Marijuana and hemp horticulture will be HUGE! Whether it be growing medical or recreational marijuana, or industrial hemp, in the coming years there will be millions of acres devoted to these crops, and thousands of new jobs created.

A degree in chemistry, especially organic chemistry, could also be a giant plus. There will be a huge need for marijuana testing laboratory personnel over the next decade. This degree plus a self-taught knowledge of marijuana would almost assure you of great employment. Of all of the possible marijuana jobs these could be the highest paying jobs of all.

WORK FOR A DISPENSARY:

If possible, assuming marijuana is legal where you live, visit some dispensaries. You will probably need a "marijuana medical card" to gain access, except in the five venues that presently allow recreational use. If you suffer from any chronic pain, as many do, it is relatively easy in most states to obtain this dispensary-entry credential.

You will see that every dispensary employs a number of specialists. It starts with the entry security and check in, to the workers behind the next security door who actually discuss and weigh and document and dispense the physical marijuana products.

There are usually two to five such individuals, each with a specific function. One usually is designated to handle the purchase transaction itself, which at present is almost always in cash.

WORK FOR A GROWER:

Marijuana grow facilities are *highly specialized* farms. Because of the complexities of growing quality marijuana it is far different from growing a crop such as wheat or corn. The grows might be indoors or outdoors. The owners need specialists in growing in soil, in water and in air. They need fertilizer specialists. They need lighting specialists. They need water distribution experts. They need HVAC (heating, ventilating and air conditioning) specialists. They need electricians. They need individuals to bar code every plant. They need individuals known as "bud tenders".

Each of these "needs" is for individuals who have the basic credentials AND have the unique knowledge peculiar to a marijuana grow facility.

Owners especially need the individuals who process the mature plants. "Bud trimming" is a particular delicate specialty, and it is a known fact that there are very few really expert bud trimmers. Learn to be one!

WORK FOR A BAKERY OR FOOD PROCESSOR:

It is a fact that over **_half_** of all revenue generated by most dispensaries is derived from all manner of edible products! This includes cakes, cookies, cupcakes and brownies. It includes chocolate specialties. It includes hard and soft candies and lollypops. It includes smoothie drinks, and carbonated drinks and "pep" drinks. Someone somewhere has to make these. It might as well be you!

What complicates the issue is where and how to you obtain the marijuana with which to infuse the products? If we are talking adding "hemp oil", that particular item is readily available legally everywhere in the United States. (All of it is imported; See Chapter 12.) You could create all manner of hemp-infused products without a marijuana supply. These could be cannabidiol rich (CBD), but would not contain THC.

However, there are two other possibilities. Many dispensaries will be running on-site facilities to create edibles. They will need a "master chef" and "bakery workers" at the dispensary site. The possibilities here are considerable.

You could also provide edibles wherein the dispensary would add their own marijuana derivatives AFTER you deliver the yummies. This addition would have to be as simple a process as possible, but surely not beyond reason.

Of course every state will have its own bureaucratic web of regulations regarding edibles, licensing fees, taxes, and everything else imaginable to make earning a living in the marijuana edibles industry as difficult and unprofitable as possible! Meddling in success is a government art form.

START A TESTING LABORATORY OR WORK IN ONE:

Virtually every state mandates testing of all marijuana products sold, both for potency and for contaminants. There will be a huge need for specialty laboratories. The start-up costs can be very high, because the equipment needed (e.g., spectrometers, DNA testers, etc.) is very expensive, but the profits could be huge.

For those who can afford a lab, it will be difficult to staff it with qualified personnel. Here again there will be state regulations. Expect the Lab Director (not necessarily the owner) to probably need a PhD in some related field. The support personnel will have to pass security muster, and probably need a chemistry degree. There may, however, be intern or trainee positions for which almost anyone without a criminal record could qualify.

WORK FOR A "CONCENTRATOR":

This is somewhat similar to a testing lab, but far more dangerous. Among the key products offered by dispensaries are "oils". These are highly concentrated THC and CBD products created from various marijuana plant materials. Some processes to create these products use highly volatile (i.e.,flammable and explosive) solvents and gases.

Fire, explosions and death are far from impossible.   As the saying goes, it's a tough job but someone has to do it! The requirements here would be quite similar to those for the testing labs.

INSURANCE AGENTS:

Don't have an insurance license? Are you semi-literate and of average intelligence? With no intention of disparaging insurance agents, I can tell you from having been insurance licensed in at least three states over the years that obtaining a license is quite easy. It is far easier than obtaining licenses for securities, real estate, and mortgages (not that any of those require a genius IQ either.)

Consider becoming licensed, preferably in a state that has license reciprocity with a lot of other states. If you already *are* licensed, great! The marijuana industry needs a LOT of insurance, and most of it is expensive insurance. (Read: "high commissions"!) Start with key-man insurance.

If a company has raised a few million dollars from an investor or investor group said investor needs positive assurance that the key individuals (usually from one to three, most often just one) do not die unexpectedly and doom the company to

225

instant extinction!

Of course fire insurance is important. Testing labs and extraction facilities would be especially critical, because they deal with highly flammable solvents. Dispensaries are petty-thief magnets. Grow facilities are professional thief and drug cartel magnets. Employee health insurance? Accident insurance? You name it, the marijuana industry needs it.

And then there is the need for protection against unimaginable and unforeseeable consequences unique to being *in* the marijuana business itself.

You show me an insurance agent who is a **TRUE** master of marijuana industry risk mitigation (one who has REALLY done his homework) and I'll show you a *very* successful insurance agent. Specialization is always the key to success.

CREATING LOTIONS AND TOPICAL CREAMS:

Remember, anyone can create products that contain CBD-rich hemp oil, which is legal everywhere in the United States. Lotions and topical creams have great potential for any creative entrepreneur.

If you want to create such products using marijuana-based derivatives, perhaps a dispensary would set aside an area within their facility where you could create these products on site.

COMPUTER SOFTWARE:

The regulated marijuana industry is based on "seed to sale" tracking. Literally every seed is bar-coded, and that tiny seed is traced right up to whatever end products are derived from the final plant. There already exists a number of software programs. Could they be improved? Simplified? Probably.

There is also an absolute nightmare of dispensary regulations and record keeping. I know from talking with a number of dispensary owners that any software that can make their lives easier is very welcome. Much software already exists, but is it the best possible? Doubtful. So you, master software guru, have an opportunity to learn the industry and develop some killer software and make your fortune!

SET UP A MARIJUANA DELIVERY COMPANY:

Many dispensaries will be delivering marijuana products directly to their patients' homes. They can't mail products…a federal no-no. FedX and UPS may not touch it. Dispensaries will be delivering marijuana products by private car. This will not be quite as easy as working for Uber. There will be major bonding and security issues. The states will govern the hell out of it as with every aspect of the marijuana industry. This is still an area very much worth exploring. Someone has to do it. Why not you?

ADDRESS SECURITY ISSUES:

There is probably no industry that is more challenged by security issues than the marijuana industry.

Dispensaries are an easy target for thieves. Not only the product, but all of that tempting cash! Are you a security-device specialist? If so, adapt your skills to the needs of marijuana dispensaries.

Grow facilities are particularly vulnerable to theft, especially outdoor facilities. Are you a security-fencing specialist? Are you a surveillance device specialist? Can you supply trained guard Dobermans? These are very real potential niche jobs in this rapidly expanding industry.

Many facilities will be hiring ex-military personnel and ex law-enforcement officers. I've seen a few dispensaries with Andre The Giant or Attila The Hun lurking outside! Being a six-foot-six seventh-degree black belt karateka body-builder type could well land you a lucrative job in marijuana security. But remember, you will be paid to *notice* things and to *prevent* problems, not to look to display your Herculean skills!

STAFFING:

"Employment Agencies" are a dime a dozen. "Marijuana Industry Specialty Employment Agencies" are, for now, very rare. This is an incredible opportunity for anyone anywhere who knows how (through internet and social media?) to create lists of employable specialists in every marijuana niche. The ability to find qualified individuals and market those individuals to the industry is a huge potential opportunity.

MARKETING, SALES, PROMOTION & COMPLIANCE CONSULTATION:

Here again is a business that can be run from anywhere. Can you create a super-effective website? BINGO! Are you a marketing or sales guru? BINGO! Just mold these skills to the industry by LEARNING THE INDUSTRY.

Don't assume the owners of various marijuana niche companies actually KNOW anything! They may (or may not) be expert in their particular marijuana niche. Even if they are do they know diddly-squat about marketing?

It has been reported that dispensary owners spend an average of *two days* a week on regulatory and compliance matters! They would rather pay YOU than DO!

Each state will have different complex, voluminous, ever-changing rules and regulations. Become an expert in a given state's rules and regulations and you could be extremely

228

valuable to any dispensary owner or grower.

DISPENSARIES AND GROW AREA JANITORS:

Don't overlook this relatively low-tech need. There are security and bonding issues that *many* applicants will be unable to pass. The pay could be decent for applicants that *can* pass muster AND show some knowledge of the industry. Especially for grow facilities, "clean up" can be an exacting endeavor requiring skill and understanding of marijuana.

BE AN INVESTOR - FINDER:

Have you had experience raising money for any company or non-profit organization? Do you know how to write an effective business plan or grant request? This is a job that can be run from your bedroom if you have a thorough understanding of investor needs and wants as they pertain to this fledgling industry.

There are literally hundreds of marijuana companies *starving* for cash. There are thousands of potential investors that are scared to death to commit capital to this federally-illegal industry. If you are good at providing this investor-finder service you could earn massive commissions.

GRAPHIC ART:

There is a real need for graphic artists' skills in the marijuana industry. Can you create a killer logo? Can you create exciting package design? How about website graphics? If you think you are good, create a portfolio of your work and see if you can market it to the hundreds of companies in the industry that you can identify with a simple Google search. One or more companies just might fall all over themselves to pay you for your graphic arts skills.

CREATE A COMIC BOOK:

229

OK, this one is a bit far-fetched. I haven't seen "The Marijuana Dude" or "Mr. SuperWeed" or "Ganja Joe" or "Sally Sinsamilla" or "The Amazing Stoner Man" yet. I'm sure I will! There are actually people out there (I've known a few) who are *really* good at this sort of thing. It might be a fun project, and you never know! It's all about marketing your skills.

PACKAGING AND LABELING:

Do you have a background in product packaging? This could be vacuum sealing, or zip lock bags, glass and plastic bottles of all kinds and sizes, or anything else that can contain an edible product, an oily liquid, a tincture, a liquid product, or raw marijuana. Can you come up with something better, easier, cheaper? This is a largely unexplored area, but very critical to the entire marijuana industry, because EVERY PRODUCT must be packaged attractively and properly.

REAL ESTATE ENDEAVORS:

A real estate license in a given state could be a big plus here. Licensing, however, may not be required for certain jobs.

For example, without a license you could be a "finder". Marijuana companies will be looking for warehouses for indoor grow facilities. They will be looking for land for outdoor grow operations. The problem is that every state will have its own Draconian regulations as to what and where and how marijuana can be grown. Learn their rules.

You don't need a license to study zoning laws. You don' need a license to be a finder-consultant. You *do* need a license to actually sell real estate for others.

There are other real estate related possibilities. Are you a landlord? You might consider "marijuana-friendly" specialty housing or apartments. How about a marijuana-friendly Bed and Breakfast? How about a "Marijuana Lounge"? Of course every state will be looking at any of these to earn ridiculously-high "licensing fees"!

CAREGIVING:

Many marijuana patients are likely to be bed-ridden. Many will need housekeeping. Many will need a dog walker. Many will need someone to shop for groceries. Perhaps you could convince a dispensary to offer your services to such individuals, a win-win for them and you. Well worth considering.

OPEN A "HEAD SHOP":

Now here is a retail business where you do not "touch the plant", and where the incredible array of products available from China and around the world is almost limitless! You can sell paraphernalia such as bongs, hookahs, vaporizers, books, t-shirts, anything marijuana except marijuana itself! You should also be able to sell CBD-rich hemp oil.

BE A MARIJUANA WRITER OR BLOGGER:

Can you write? Can you blog? If so, there are endless possibilities within the industry.

Why not start a *state-specific* magazine? None exist at present as far I know. Aside from potential subscription revenue, advertising revenue from almost every marijuana-related company in the state could be huge!

You could also publish a series of subject-specific books or booklets. Marijuana cookbooks, although there are many already in print, sell well. You could create state and local lists of marijuana-friendly professionals, doctors, lawyers, etc. You could research and publish compendiums of current marijuana research. This area is limited only by your imagination.

Are you are an experienced blogger? Do you know how to promote anything via Facebook, Pinterest, You Tube, LinkedIn or Twitter? If so, your talents should be in **GREAT** demand. Most owners of the hundreds of public companies are forty to sixty years old and were *not* brought up in the social media culture. Many have *zero* knowledge in these areas and would absolutely kill to have an effective blog set up on their website or develop effective social communication. Big potential here.

The problem here is that you may be walking a fine legal line. Enormous companies such as Facebook, Twitter and Google feel that it will tarnish their reputation if they allow overt marijuana advertising. This should change in the future. It will take creative article writing to get around their restrictions.

BE AN INDEPENDENT- CONTRACTOR PUBLIC-SPEAKER:

There have been studies that show many people fear public speaking more than death! A root canal (double nerve) is always considered a better choice. Yet there are some, either by nature or formal training who are totally comfortable in front of an audience. These people can command outrageous speaking fees!

Every marijuana convention has speakers that attendees pay big bucks to hear. They represent companies in every imaginable niche in the industry. Some speakers are company employees, but MANY are hired independent-contractor speakers.

If you have speaking skills, or are willing to acquire them, AND you learn the industry, you may well be able to advertise your skills to the hundreds of companies who exhibit and attend these frequent conferences. You could land some regular all-expense-paid visits to great locations all around the country and get paid handsomely for your time as well!

CREATE A *LOCAL* CANNABIS CONFERENCE YOURSELF:

Study the many huge regional marijuana conferences. Learn who attends, how they advertise, what they charge exhibitors and attendees. Consider creating a state-specific scaled-down version. This might not be as hard as it sounds! It can be tied in with advertising, and even with local hotel bookings and travel arrangements. From what I have been told this can be a huge money-maker.

PAYMENT PROCESSING:

Can you tackle the one major problem for the medical marijuana industry: payments. It's still a cash-based industry. Many buyers do not want marijuana transactions on their regular credit cards. Very few banks are willing to have a medical marijuana company appearing in their records. Can someone out there create a special marijuana credit card? Can someone perhaps start a marijuana-exclusive non-government-insured bank? It can be done.

EXCHANGE-TRADED SECURITIES TRACKING AND REPORTING:

There will be eventually thousands of companies involved in some aspect of the marijuana industry. Many will be listed on one of the stock exchanges. There will be a need for a publication that tracks the progress of individual companies and their stocks. Quarterly reports are public information. Investors will be eager to find detailed information compiled in one place. Could you create such a publication?

GOVERNMENT JOBS:

Legalization will create MANY more government jobs. For example, because it is easy for drug cartels to plant their marijuana seedlings inside of a large legal grow facility there will be a whole new *army* of federal Agents. These specialists will have the dangerous job of checking crops and testing plants to identify strains that differ from the intended legal crop. Of course if the illicit crop is the exact same strain as the legal crop this creates a different problem unto itself.

There will also be an army of new federal and state inspectors needed. They will be inspecting grow facilities, testing laboratories, dispensaries and head shops. These should all be well-paying long-term positions with great benefits and retirement pensions.

On the other hand, this can be a very dangerous profession. In Hawaii it is well known that inspectors looking for illegal crops in remote locations have been known to go in and never reappear! This is primarily why so much marijuana is grown illegally in the Islands. No one dares to intercede in many remote areas. It *can* be fatal!

PUBLIC RELATIONS:

Do you have public relations experience? For marijuana companies hiring a public relations firm can be a major headache. Even companies that do not "touch the plant" often get rejected. The usual social channels, Google, Apple, Facebook and Instagram allow absolutely NO direct marijuana-related marketing or sales at the present time. This will change in the future as legalization advances nationwide.

LIGHTING:

Do you have any knowledge of solar power? If so, the

marijuana growing industry might have a place for you in the future. Special lighting is critical to all indoor growing operations. Electricity actually accounts for up to 50% of the wholesale cost of marijuana! Every grower needs to reduce electrical costs as much as possible. Teach them how!

In summary, I believe the most important qualities anyone contemplating employment in this new industry are knowledge and PASSION. You must be passionate about helping those in medical need. You must be passionate about the good that recreational marijuana use can bring to society. You must want to learn ***everything*** you can about this wonderful curing herb.

Once you *feel* the passion, and embark on a serious learning experience, you will be in a far better position to earn a great living in this exciting, exploding new industry.

CHAPTER 33
THE BIG CASINO –
DO RICHES AWAIT?

ARE MARIJUANA INDUSTRY INVESTORS
BRAVE OR STUPID?

Richard Branson, **Founder & Chairman of Virgin Group:**
"Decriminalization does not result in increased drug use.
Portugal's ten year experiment shows clearly that enough
is enough. It is time to end the war on drugs worldwide.
We must stop criminalizing drug users. Health and
treatment should be offered to drug users - not prison.
Bad drugs policies affect literally hundreds of thousands
of individuals and communities across the world. We
need to provide medical help to those that have
problematic use - not criminal retribution."

In writing this Chapter I am taking a risk. I've never been
sued for anything; I'd hate to start now! Of course my
attorney provided the required "boiler plate" disclaimers, but
some pissed-off corporate executive might not be overjoyed at
what I might mention below about their shaky stock.

First off, let me explain my qualifications for even touching on
this topic. I was *directly* involved in Wall Street for over thirty
years. I was a General Securities *Principal*, and a Municipal
Securities *Principal*, a very rare combination of licenses.

For many years I worked at two famous "wire houses", Dean
Witter Reynolds and Smith Barney Harris Upham. I worked
for a conservative regional firm, Advest. My wife and I had
our own Office of Supervisory Jurisdiction (OSJ), The
Investment Center. I even worked for the micro-cap firm

Stratton Oakmont performing nationwide outside-company due diligence studies for Jordan Belfort, the infamous *Wolf of Wall Street* himself. This was long before government intervention shut him down for money laundering.

I won top awards at the wire houses (e.g., #1 in the hyper-competitive New York City market; #7 nationally). Throughout my Wall Street career (from which I voluntarily retired a few years ago) and tens of thousands of transactions I had an extremely clean compliance record. There were just two minor silly complaints, both resolved in my favor!

How do I define "silly"? How about a CPA who complained he did not understand his monthly statements? Or a couple who decided I should pay for their Island vacation because they couldn't find an investment they wanted? Incredible.

I was (and still am) a Registered Financial Planner. I have held top level executive positions in three Fortune 500 Divisions, and started a number of companies as an entrepreneur, some successful, some not. I have navigated Chapter 11 reorganizations and Chapter 7 dissolutions.

I have been on the Boards of Directors of a number of stock exchange listed companies. I was Chief Operating Officer and Corporate Secretary of Judicate, The National Private Court System, during its formative years. **In short, I've been around the financial block more than a few times!**

I've written and analyzed dozens of corporate quarterly and annual reports. I'm pretty good at spotting strengths and weaknesses, and calculating the key financial ratios.

Does this extensive background make me an "expert" at anything? Not at all. But it does give me more financial experience than most persons evaluating companies from both outside and inside. I have seen what works and what does not work. I have seen how companies lie to their investors and manipulate financial facts. I have learned to believe nothing unless I am an actual party to it. **Nothing.**

For the past five years I have carefully studied the emerging marijuana market. I believe I own or have read every book ever written on the subject. I subscribe to every marijuana newsletter I can find, and spend at least an hour a day reading any industry reports available on line. In *great* moderation I buy the stocks of some companies in the marijuana field, ONLY with money I can <u>totally afford to lose.</u>

Remember the "dot com bubble"? There was a dizzying number of under-capitalized startup companies with seemingly great ideas. Most of their young executives had very little executive experience in running *anything*, let alone a corporation. Collapse was inevitable. Collapse happened.

How does that compare with the infant marijuana industry? In my opinion, they are very similar in many ways. They are *very* different in others. Many of the dot-com ideas were "virtual". There was nothing in the way of physical product involved in most cases. They were selling hot air, smoke and mirrors. There were many great sounding ideas with no past experience to accurately predict future performance.

In contrast, the marijuana industry has a wide variety of *physical* products. There is the marijuana plant itself, all of the derivatives from the plant (oils, tinctures, edibles, etc.), all of the delivery equipment (vaporizers, bongs), and all of the growing equipment (special lights, solar panels). There are the "virtual" items, tracking software, consulting, tax and legal work. There are the important testing laboratories as well.

There are two very different "divisions" of the marijuana industry. There are the companies that "<u>touch the plant</u>", and those that "do *not* <u>touch the plant</u>". It is a *very* important distinction because they are taxed and regulated differently by the feds and by the states.

There is the one inconvenient way that the marijuana industry differs from the dot com industry. It certainly does not favor the marijuana industry at this time. **Marijuana is illegal on the federal level.** Why does this matter?
- Banks are unwilling or unable to handle money generated by marijuana companies;
- It is virtually impossible to get bank loans;
- It is virtually impossible to get credit cards or a credit line;
- Business expenses are **not federally tax deductible** in many cases;
- The entire marijuana industry is overwhelmed with costly seed-to-sale tracking regulations at the state level;
- If the "wrong" United States president gets elected the entire industry could be shut down **completely**!

Perhaps even more important is the fact that the entire marijuana industry is competing against the six hundred pound gorilla in the room, **THE CARTELS.** Unhampered by regulations, and generally ruthless in their business practices, having to play the game by the government's rules puts the entire legal marijuana industry at a serious disadvantage.

So, no matter how well funded, no matter how well managed, companies in this specialized marijuana business sector face many barriers to profitability. This includes the threat of total extinction that the dot coms did not ever face. Most of *them* failed anyway!

There is one primary reason **ANY** company in **ANY** industry fails: **UNDER-CAPITALIZATION!** I don't care how great management is, I don't care how great a product or idea is, if the company does not have the cash to fund its startup phase, and carry itself through to profitability, it simply dies. The death can be rapid. The death can be painfully slow. Either way the principal, investors and stockholders are screwed.

Most companies in the marijuana industry are in *desperate* need of cash. Thanks to Uncle Sam they cannot get it from conventional sources, so they must get it from "angel" investors (private wealthy folks) or from Hedge Funds. The problem here is that this sort of private capital is **very hard to come by.** When you do find it, it is very costly.

Wealthy investors, and successful Hedge Funds, are wealthy and successful for two reasons. They are very smart, and they are very cautious.

With all of the above said, there are *well over a hundred* publically-traded marijuana companies and countless other privately held marijuana companies, all competing in an industry that is **federally illegal**. Not exactly a great fundamental business model for success!

Since 1978 when I became directly involved in Wall Street I have seen the stock market rise and fall like a roller coaster. I've seen fortunes made and lost. I've seen at least two "major market corrections". I have never been a "stock-jock", defined in the industry as a broker who focuses on helping his clients outsmart the markets. I contend that the latter is impossible. It is worse than a casino!

I have always considered the stock market to be the "Big Casino", and I have referred to it as such in books I've written that go back decades. My focus as a broker was always on selling high quality municipal bonds, and government-backed securities. I didn't get as rich as many other brokers, but my clients didn't get poor either! It is hard to believe, but when I was first involved in the markets government insured bank CDs were paying up to 21%. Today it is impossible to find one paying 2%! Times they are a'changin!

I can recall selling AAA rated General Obligation U.S. state bonds at 16%! The low interest rates today are one reason so many of our seniors are struggling to make ends meet. But that's a story for another book.

There is an amusing story that goes back a century or so. J. Pierpont Morgan was the wealthiest man in America. He was so wealthy he even bailed out the United States Treasury once when they were short of funds! Old J.P. would never give out the secrets of his continual investing success.

One investor finally prevailed. He offered Morgan $50,000, a huge sum in those days, for a sit-down session to learn Morgan's closely guarded secrets. The meeting lasted one minute, and consisted of four words from Morgan: "Buy Low. Sell High"! Simple, to the point, and as on-target as one could possibly get.

Warren Buffet, today's rough equivalent of J. P. Morgan, has one basic investing philosophy. Before investing in a company he believes one MUST acquire in-depth knowledge of the <u>INDUSTRY</u>. Only then should one begin to acquire in depth knowledge of a particular company within that industry. If you do not thoroughly understand the workings of a given industry and how all the competitors interact you cannot even *begin* to evaluate a given company correctly.

The markets today are so very different from when I entered the industry that they are unrecognizable. Very few investors realize that over 90% of all stock market trades today are made by <u>robot investing programs</u>! Zero human interaction.

The timing of trades is so precise and critical that one company recently paid hundreds of thousands of dollars to set up a fiber-optics system that would gain them a *seven-millisecond* advantage! Anyone who believes they can compete effectively in the stock market today is nuts.

With that said, speculators today have a great advantage over those of a few decades ago. The internet allows anyone to research companies in ways that were once impossible . For starters, drill down into any company website and gain a real understanding of what they do and how they do it. You will often also see short biographies of the management team.

THEN access the company's latest Annual Report, and the latest Quarterly Reports. This is greatly facilitated if you have an on-line stock brokerage account such as Ameritrade.

It helps to know what to look for! It is pretty easy to see whether a company has any money, makes any sales, and even might (SURPRISE!) show a profit! You can study these reports and find all of the legal "dirt", possible lawsuits and the like that can adversely affect a company long term.

All of which brings me to the reason for this Chapter on marijuana-related public companies. There are dozens of these stocks from which to choose. The dream of getting in on the ground floor of a truly successful company is hard to resist for many individuals. Every IBM was a low-cost start-up stock somewhere along the line.

Americans spend zillions of dollars on lottery tickets with a five-hundred-million-plus to one chances of winning. The odds of scoring big on a speculative marijuana stock should be at least that good! What seasoned speculative investor can resist buying a million shares of a stock, *any* stock, for a thousand bucks, and sometimes for much less?

This is especially true for a "penny" marijuana stock that may at some time in the past been over a dollar and with luck (read "financing") sometime in the future might even exceed that!

So how do you choose which marijuana "dog" to toss a few bones at? Some serious internet research is not a bad idea.

Every listed company must disclose the identity of its executives. There are any number of on-line companies that offer "people search" websites where you can literally find out ANYTHING about anyone, for a modest fee. You can often identify the executives from their websites. You can *always* identify them from the periodic documents the stock exchanges require them to file.

For starters, after you have studied the website propaganda of a company in which you are considering investing and find it interesting, try checking out the past history of its top executives! Be sure you are sitting down. Some backgrounds can be pretty ugly! Many are not so awful.

It's not a bad idea to call the company and talk with executives as high up the ladder as possible. If you are comfortable fibbing a bit, if you pretend to be a big time investor or start-up seed money angel you can probably get in touch with the head honcho in a flash. The promise of ready investment capital can open many otherwise-closed doors!

The physical appearance of the corporate websites themselves can tell you a lot. A really crappy looking website (or none at all) is a pretty good indicator of what one might expect from any company. Crap, or nothing! I immediately eliminate from speculation consideration any company without a really decent website.

Then of course look at the company's published financials, assuming they have been around long enough to even *have* financials. Have they been able to borrow money? As I said earlier, the death knell of any company is under-capitalization.

Even if they *have* managed to find an angel "hard-money" investor because conventional investing is unavailable, you can be certain they are paying 12% to 14% or more for the loan. This can have a huge effect on future profitability. Can they afford this major monthly interest expense long term?

Did they have to give up a huge percentage of the company to raise the money? If possible, see if anyone in authority with whom you manage to speak can give you a hint of whether the "angel" is more of a "Devil" in terms of meddling with day to day operations. They often are.

Combine the high cost of borrowing with all of the other normal business costs and you can see clearly that only those marijuana companies with top quality management and a viable business plan and/or a unique product have a **prayer** of long-term survival.

So here is where I put my neck out and discuss a few companies that I follow that I think might have *some* chance of survival. This is not to say that there are not hundreds of better companies with better prospects. Nor is it to say that investing in any of these is a particularly good idea. It isn't.

THE *ENTIRE* MARIJUANA INDUSTRY AT THIS TIME MUST BE CONSIDERED *HIGHLY SPECULATIVE* . ONLY INVEST MONEY IN THIS INDUSTRY THAT YOU CAN

**AFFORD TO LOSE WITHOUT SO MUCH AS BLINKING!
THIS IS PURE GAMBLING. THE BIG CASINO IN SPADES.**

I have not received anything at all in the way of compensation from any of these companies nor do I personally know any of the executives involved (WEED, Inc. excepted). In fact, if I were investing *large* sums of money in any of these I would VISIT the company physically before investing. That is always a good idea. *I am absolutely certain that some exchange-listed marijuana companies are being run out of the CEO's garage or basement!*

As mentioned above, in the marijuana industry there are two very basic categories. The separator is whether or not they **"touch the plant"**. This is a huge distinction, because those who are "touching the plant" have far more barriers to success than those who do not "touch the plant". Remember, however, that even though a company may not touch the plant, they are still dependent on the fundamental success of the industry as a whole.

DISCLAIMER: (In addition to the legalese at the beginning of the book.) Neither the author nor anyone connected in any way with this book assumes any liability for any losses sustained by any investor. These are not "buy" recommendations nor "sell" recommendations nor "hold" recommendations. They are not recommendations of any kind. It is a compilation of public information offered as such.

The author may or may not hold a position in any of these stocks. We wish to emphasize that no sane and honest investment advisor would recommend putting one cent into this industry, at least until the federal government decriminalizes and un-schedules or re-schedules marijuana to Schedule III or better. Any one of these companies is pure speculation. Any investment should be with money that you can <u>absolutely afford to lose</u>.

NOTE: Canadian companies are operating under a totally different environment, because the Canadian government is far more enlightened then ours. The problem they have that we do not have is that they have <u>far fewer</u> potential users. Canada has a total population of only 36,000,000 vs the United States with upwards of 350,000,000 citizens (counting those in the country illegally.)

Of course the *entire* stock market can be influenced dramatically by events that are unforeseen. The sudden death of a President. A massive terrorist attack on home soil. The loss of the power grid for an extended time. A collapse of the monetary system. A massive correction (6,000 points+?) in the stock market. This is one reason why investing <u>in *any* stock in *any* market</u> is *always* a gamble. It is why I refer to all the markets as "The Big Casino"!

You will not find the marijuana public companies listed any time soon on the New York Stock Exchange! You will find them on the huge "Over The Counter" (OTC) markets. There are almost ten thousand companies that trade "Over The Counter", a hundred-plus of these in the marijuana business.

I say "market<u>s</u>", plural, because there are three distinct OTC marketplaces.

Most of the under-capitalized, newly minted marijuana public companies trade on the **"OTC Pink Sheets"**. (The term "Pink Sheets" derives from the fact that in the pre-internet days there was a published printed list of all of the stocks presented in this market, and it was printed on pink colored paper.)

There are many fine companies on the Pink Sheets, including some in business for decades. Do not ever ignore a company simply because it is listed in this marketplace. Within the Pink Sheets there are three subcategories. These are: "Current information", "Limited information" and "No information", based on the most recent filing deadlines.

The "information" referred to is the current financial data. Some companies may simply be late in their filings, but all else may be fine. Even those with "no reporting" may not necessarily be bad companies. There can be many extenuating circumstances that delay timely reporting.

The other two OTC marketplaces are the QB and QX. The **OTCQB** is referred to as "The Venture Marketplace". It is intended for entrepreneurial and development-stage companies. This is the trading arena where you will find the majority of marijuana company stocks listed.

The **OTCQX** is the *elite* area of the OTC markets. It is only for those companies that are current in their reporting, meet high financial standards, and receive third-party advisory. This is not to imply that these companies necessarily have any better chance of long-range success than any others on the QB or Pink Sheets.

You will also find a few companies that are publically traded, but NOT on the OTC. These are the **"Gray Market"** (often written "Grey") stocks, completely unregulated, but legal. If you are considering any of these it would be particularly wise to do extensive due diligence.

Please again note I am NOT making any sort of recommendation or prediction relative to the stocks on my list. This is all public information. It is a random sample of companies I am interested in following in order to get some gauge of how different marijuana market segments might be progressing.

I strongly urge anyone who is considering speculating in any of these stocks to do complete due diligence on their own. For a website that tracks over eighty such companies check out: marijuanastocks.com. All of the figures below are correct as of the moment I am writing this Chapter. There will certainly be many changes by the time you read this book.

In studying the following stock information, note that:

$0.5000 is fifty cents/share, $1.00/2 shares, $1,000/2,000 shares;

$0.1000 is ten cents/share, $1.00/10 shares, $1,000/10,000 shares;

$0.0100 is one penny/share, $1.00/100 shares, $1,000/ 100,000 shares (the classic "penny stock");

$0.0010 is 1/10th penny/share, $1.00/1,000 shares, $1,000/ 1 million shares;

$0.00010 is 1/100th penny/share, $1.00/10,000 shares, $1,000/ 10 million shares. What a bargain! (???)

To calculate what percentage of a company's outstanding shares you own, divide the shares you own by the shares outstanding.

Incidentally, the common vernacular within the securities industry for these very cheap stocks is "shit kickers"! More politely they are generally classified as "penny stocks". Here is a list of twenty-one among those I follow that qualify:

Blue Line Protection Group, Inc. (BLPG: OTC Pink/Limited info.) Offer protection and transportation services. Latest year: $0.012 - $0.135. (All-time high $1.10+.) Current: $0.054. Shares outstanding: 125 million.

Cannabix Technologies, Inc. (BLOZF: OTC Pink/Current info.) Latest year: $0.08 - $0.30. Current: $0.225. Shares outstanding: 63 million.

CV Sciences, Inc. (CANV: OTCQB) Latest year: $0.10 - $1.80. Current: $0.490. Shares outstanding: 52 million.

Enertopia Corp. (ENRT: OTCQB) Renewal energy, oil & gas, medical marijuana. Developmental stage. Latest year: $.0055 – 0.04 (All-time high $0.80). Current $0.020. Canadian. Shares outstanding: 72 million.

Growblox Sciences (GBLX: OTCQB) Conversion of marijuana into useful products. Latest year: $0.11 - $0.74, Current $0.190. (All-time high $3.50+) Shares outstanding: 46 million.

Hemp, Inc. (HEMP: OTC Pink/Current info.) Great name and symbol! Hemp products. Latest year: $.025 - $1.00. Current: 0.050. Shares outstanding 2.1 billion.

Kaya Holdings, Inc. (KAYS: OTCQB) A holding company. Own a marijuana dispensary. Latest year: $0.045 - $0.150. Current: $0.060. Shares outstanding: 89 million.

Kush Bottles, Inc. (KSHB: OTCQB) Latest year: $0.70 - $10.00. Current: $1.13. Shares outstanding: 47 million.

Marijuana Company of America, Inc. (MCOA: OTC Pink/Current info.) Distributor of marijuana products. Latest year: $0.002 - $0.030. Current: $0.011. Shares outstanding: 47 million.

Mass Roots, Inc. (MSRT: OTCQB) A marijuana social

network. Latest year: $0.65 - $2.34. Current: $1.00. Shares outstanding: 48 million.

mCig, Inc. (MCIG: OTCQB) Electronic marijuana cigarettes. Latest year: $.018 - $.09. Current: $0.038. Shares outstanding: 301 million.

Medical Marijuana, Inc. (MJNA: OTC Pink/Current info.) Highly diversified into many marijuana markets. Latest year: $0.0275 - $0.115. Current: 0.050. Shares outstanding: 1.8 billion.

Medican Enterprises, Inc. (MDCN: OTC Pink/No info.) A bio-pharmaceutical company. Latest year: $0.0001 - $0.0150. Current: $0.0001. Shares outstanding: 2.6 billion.

Orgenesis, Inc. (ORGS: OTCQB) Cell-based studies. Latest year: $0.235 - $0.620. Current: $0.380. Shares outstanding: 109 million.

Pineapple Express, Inc. (PNPL: Gray Market – Caution!) Latest year: $0.02 - $42.30. (All time high: $150.00!) Current: $9.15. Shares outstanding: 54 million.

Strainwise, Inc. (STWC: OTC Pink/Current info.) Branding, marketing and administrative services. Recently involved with Native Americans. Latest year: $0.410 - $1.00. Current: $0.470. Shares outstanding: 27 million.

Supreme Pharmaceuticals, Inc. (SPRWF: OTC Pink/Current info.) Latest Year: $0.080 - $0.450 (All-time high at $0.710). Current: $0.290. Canadian. Shares outstanding: 98 million.

Surna, Inc. (SRNA: OTCQB) Indoor climate control systems. Latest Year: $0.040 - $0.250. Current $0.080. Shares outstanding: 139 million.

Terra Tech Corp. (TRTC: OTCQX) A holding company. Into

hydroponics. Latest year $0.080 – 0.750. Current: $0.410. Shares outstanding: 344 million.

Two Rivers Water and Farming Co. (TURV: OTCQB) Acquires farmland and water rights. Latest Year: $0.250 - $1.10 (All-time high $2.95), current $0.360. Shares outstanding: 27 million.

WEED, Inc. (BUDZ: OTC Pink/No info.) Great name and stock symbol! Highly diversified into many possible marijuana markets. Seeking capital. Latest year: $0.043 - $0.150. Current: $0.060. Shares outstanding: 14 million. (NOTE: I am a paid engineering consultant and writer for this company.)

Worldwide Diversified Holdings, Inc. (WNTR: OTC Pink/Current info.) Latest year: $0.0001 - $0.0003. (All-time high: $0.300.) Latest: $0.0001.

The most extraordinary thing about the above stocks (*not* chosen to show this aspect) is the *enormous* range in price during the past year and in some cases from the all-time high. This is typical of almost *all* stocks in the marijuana industry.

Prices tend to jump on almost ANY positive news, then slide back waiting for the next "exciting" corporate announcement. There is no way to know how accurate or honest these announcements actually are. I suspect many are fiction!

I know one investor who day-trades penny stocks. He follows a small list of under-a-dollar stocks. He looks for consistent daily up and down trends, and "Buys Low, Sells High". With today's extraordinarily low cost investor trades a tiny move in a penny stock can equate to a big profit depending on the size of the trade. Compared to decades ago the trading costs are almost like having a Stock Exchange seat and free trades!

Keep this in mind. A change in a marijuana stock price from $0.0001 to $0.001 is the same percentage equivalent as IBM going from $149 to $1,490.00! **THIS** is what makes speculating in the marijuana sector so inviting, and so much fun! If you can treat "investing" in this sector as a fun hobby and a pure gamble, and participate with money you don't care if you lose, I say **"GO FOR IT"! It can be exciting.**

Of course every penny-stock "bucket shop" (I know there are some still out there) and scam artist (think Bernie Madoff) will be "pumping and dumping" low cost possibly worthless marijuana stocks. **Buyer beware!**

As a potential marijuana stock speculator there are two more factors you might wish to consider, "**corruption**" and "**preemption**". The amount of **corruption** in American businesses in general is not often discussed, but it happens in many sectors. It seems to me that the marijuana business, with its endless licensing decisions (who gets what and when) and inspections from seed to sale will be a fertile hunting ground for the unscrupulous. *Corruption is inevitable.*

When I first arrived in Hawaii I in the '90s I researched the home building industry. I had been involved in building and rehabbing homes stateside for many years, and had a pretty good idea of the various hoops one could expect to jump through for various licenses, inspections and approvals. This is not at all unlike today's marijuana industry.

One builder who had been on the Islands for many years asked me quite seriously: "Do you have a good supply of envelopes?" I wasn't quite sure what he meant. "Envelopes?" I replied. "You know, for bribes. That's the only way you will ever get anything accomplished around here." Welcome to Alohaland!

Could this sort of corrupt behavior begin to taint the young marijuana industry? Well, guess what? <u>It already has!</u> Here is a case in point:

Have A Heart Compassionate Care has four medical marijuana dispensaries and three recreational marijuana shops in Washington state. According to trial records and testimony, an IRS Agent in Seattle was assigned to audit their corporate taxes in the summer of 2015.

After conducting the audit, the IRS Agent indicated to the owner that he had saved him "millions of dollars"....but then asked him for a $20,000 bribe to "overlook" possible problems. The dispensary owner and his attorney reported the bribe request to the FBI.

The FBI then asked that the owner meet with the Agent while wearing a wire and go through with the bribe with marked bills. Result: The jury found the IRS Agent guilty....he should be out of prison around 2031, some $250,000 poorer!

There can be huge sums of money in the balance based on who is awarded a prized grow license, who is awarded a prized dispensary license, and who can establish a testing lab, a concentration facility, or an edibles operation. These licenses are eagerly sought after and worth their weight in gold. Fertile grounds for corruption? You decide.

Whether long-term corruption could have a serious major negative impact on the industry overall remains to be seen. It could certainly affect any given company caught bypassing the laws.

Preemption, on the other hand, is a reality that must eventually be resolved. This is a VERY dirty word in the marijuana industry. There is a KEY legal case in the Arizona

Courts (White Mountain Health Center, Sun City vs Maricopa County). The case dates back to 2012. The County argues that federal law **preempts** Arizona law. The county wants marijuana to be permanently outlawed, at least in *its* county.

This case is REAL, and could set a deadly precedent. Appellate Court Judge Don Kessler has gone on record as stating: "Whatever you are doing, you cannot violate federal law." Hopefully it will have been settled in favor of legalization by the time you are reading this.

The best defense against preemption is the 10th Amendment to The Constitution. It states that: "The powers not given to the federal government by The Constitution, and not prohibited by it to the states, will belong to the states." The federal government cannot force a state to criminalize private behavior. Or can they?

This matter could eventually go before the United States Supreme Court. Should a VERY conservative individual be appointed to the one presently-open bench seat, the entire industry could be doomed!

In a similar lawsuit, Nebraska and Kansas, seeing its citizens flooding into Colorado to obtain marijuana, sued Colorado. They asserted that federal law has supremacy over state law and is thereby preempted it. Fortunately they lost the case! We can only hope for the same outcome in Arizona, and that it never reaches the United States Supreme Court.

From an investing standpoint, there is the "picks and shovels" market. It may be larger than the direct "touch the plant" market. First, there is the entire agricultural sector. This affects land sales and values, as well as warehouse and greenhouse specialists. It includes specialty lighting and

254

ventilation, solar power, massive security issues requiring devices and personnel, and all manner of consulting services.

There are even many "marijuana attorneys" presently advertising their specialty! There is a large market segment related to the eclectic mix of devices for delivering the benefits of marijuana to the user. There is even a growing market for novelty items such as tee-shirts and bumper stickers! You can seek out stocks in most of these arenas.

There are about 17 million adults in the five authorities (Alaska, Colorado, District of Columbia, Oregon and Washington) where marijuana is also legal for *recreational* purposes. Looking at demographics, there are approximately 250 million *adults* in the United States. At present 135 million live in the 24 political authorities (23 states plus D.C.) where medical marijuana is legal for many different ailments.

It is reported that there are only about 1.5 million adults in the United States who presently have medical marijuana authorization cards. The present number of *legal* recreational users is impossible to know with certainty. It is conservatively estimated at a minimum of an additional 1.5 million adults. Thus, at this time, the overall *legal* marijuana market is probably around three million adults.

The *theoretical* eventual medical and recreational marijuana market is huge. No one has a real clue HOW huge. Many are predicting $100 billion in sales or higher by 2020! Because of the reluctance of most doctors to prescribe medical marijuana over Big Pharmas' heavily-promoted drugs, the ultimate marijuana market has barely been tapped.

Consider these medical statistics derived from a simple Google search:

- 21 million in the US have some form of arthritis or chronic pain;
- It is reported that there are at least 1.5 million suffering PTSD veterans (and let us not forget the 5,000+ yearly perhaps-preventable veteran suicides);
- 540,000 in the US have multiple sclerosis;
- 20 million have some sort of neuropathic pain or muscle spasms;
- 3 million suffer from glaucoma;
- 5 million+ suffer from cancer (750,000 new cases/year) and most need nausea control;
- 3 million are epileptic;
- 30,000 suffer from ALS (Lou Gehrig's Disease);
- 1.6 million have Crohn's Disease;
- 1.0 million have AIDS.

Patients suffering from all of the above diseases, and others, have been extensively reported to be helped to some extent (many *dramatically* so) by using marijuana products.

Not accounting for malady-overlap, the above amounts to 56 million+ potential *medical* marijuana patients throughout the United States! That's a lot of marijuana! So even if we never get to the point of universal recreational legalization, the potential medical marijuana market alone is huge.

It is reported that in 2014 the overall marijuana industry was worth two billion dollars ($2,000,000,000)! I have seen future estimates that vary widely, from $10 billion to over $100 billion in just four short years. Remember, it could always be **zero** (think "Chris Christie"). There are so many factors that any estimate is nothing more than a wild guess at best.

Although the potential dollar sales figures for the overall marijuana industry in the future are very compelling, there are many long-term negative forces that must be considered. Marijuana industry stocks are all *very* speculative.

Aside from the federal government, Big Pharma and other lobbies, and a corrupt media, even after a state decides on legalization there are many problems being experienced. There have been serious growing pains (unintended pun).

Dispensary licensing rules have often been virtually impossible to comply with. Action on dispensary applications can be delayed for many months or more. Taxing authorities wrestle with the issue of taxing medical and recreational uses differently. Growers are faced with all manner of stifling regulations.

The quantity of marijuana plants that legal patients are permitted to grow depends upon the licensing authority, and varies widely between states. Permitted public use outside of the home also depends upon venue.

As with any fledgling industry it is expected that all of these issues will *eventually* be resolved, but it will clearly not happen overnight. *Every problem in every sector affects the overall market in marijuana penny stocks.*

Easily overlooked is the huge area of advertising. Public marijuana advertising is illegal at this time. The internet won't touch it. Print media cannot. There are, however, little cracks in this market segment that are beginning to appear.

The huge multi-national Corporation General Mills has run ads on Colorado billboards and in media *piggybacking* on the

257

success of marijuana. On local billboards their "Totinos Pizza Rolls" were offered as a "perfect snack for 4/20 parties!" Can "Weedies" cereal be far behind? Can Super Bowl ads for marijuana products be in sight? Advertising, once it is permitted, can have a massive effect on the marijuana industry in general and on stock prices in particular.

Legally-grown marijuana wholesale prices can exceed $2,000 a pound, and retail around double that, depending upon where you live. Illegal street-marijuana often sells for half of that! This disparity-model may be the long-term downfall of the entire legal marijuana industry.

There is a major "Gold Rush of '16" well in progress, and patent attorneys are drooling! In 2015 the very first private - entity United States Patent was granted for a new marijuana strain high in THC. (Patent #9095554). New patent applications are flooding in at a record pace!

Marijuana Business Daily Conference and Exposition May 9-11 in Orlando, Florida attracted in excess of 3,000 attendees (shelling out $1,000 each at least) to see upwards of 300 exhibitors! The Gold Rush is on!

On "Marijuana Day" April 20, 2016 it is reported that marijuana retailers sold $37.5million worth of marijuana products, up 30% over that date in 2015!

Did you know that the federal government actually patented their *own* marijuana product? A private company, Kannalife Sciences, currently holds an exclusive license with the National Institute of Health (NIH) for the commercialization of a ***federal patent*** (patent #6630507)! The patent is titled: "Cannabinoids as Antioxidants and Neuroprotectants".

A Schedule I drug actually patented by Uncle Sam? **The hypocrisy of our government boggles the mind.**

To summarize, we are in a "marijuana bubble", not unlike the "dot com bubble" of a few years ago. There are over a hundred publically traded marijuana-related companies already listed. Many more are privately held. The vast majority are OTC traded penny stocks. Most are managed by individuals with little or no background in this complex industry. Many have no clear business plan. Most have zero sales and very little capital. Few will survive long term.

The key dynamic that I hope to make very clear in this Chapter is "**Buyer Beware**". The marijuana stock market is highly speculative for a large number of reasons. The long-term survival of the entire industry, much less any individual company, is not at all assured.

The federal government holds the key to the long-range success of the marijuana industry. They alone hold the key to the entire banking and private funding industries, and can unlock the door with the stroke of a pen....or shut it permanently.

If you have some extra cash and want to buy a "marijuana lottery ticket" or two, investing in this interesting new and unique industry can be a lot of fun!

You never know.

You might just hit the jackpot!

CHAPTER 34
DO BLACK LIVES *EVER* MATTER?

<u>Ed Koch</u>, Former Mayor of New York:
"In 1977, I was the principal congressional sponsor in the House of Representatives of legislation that created the National Commission on Marijuana and Drug Abuse. The commission recommended decriminalization for personal use and possession of marijuana in a limited amount. Let's stop making criminals out of our young men and women, giving them criminal records which will prevent them from getting jobs and ruin their lives."

<u>Oliver Stone</u>, Academy Award-Winning Director:
"It can be done legally, safely, healthy, and it can be taxed and the government can pay for education and stuff like that. Also, you can save a fortune by not putting kids in jail... In the black community, it is a form of slavery, this drug war, because it imprisons a huge portion of people, destroys their lives, coarsens our culture. And why?"

<u>Penn Jillette</u>, Illusionist of "Penn & Teller":
"Do we believe, even for a second, that if Obama had been busted for marijuana -- under the laws that he condones -- would his life have been better? If Obama had been caught with the marijuana that he says he used, and 'maybe a little blow'... If he had been busted under his laws...he would have done hard time... He would not be president of the United States of America. People who smoke marijuana must be set free. It is insane to lock people up."

Do black lives *ever* matter? Apparently not to our federal government and President Obama if one is considering the damage done to the lives of countless black youths for simple possession or sale of small amounts of marijuana. Thank you Uncle Sam. Thank you President Obama.

The disparity in states, counties and cities nationwide between arrest rates of black youths and white youths for possession of marijuana is enormous! Taken from the FBI's Uniform Crime Reporting Program Data and U.S. Census Data: "Nationwide blacks are almost FOUR TIMES more likely to be arrested than whites for this trivial victimless crime".

In some states, the disparity is far greater. In Iowa, Minnesota, Illinois, Kentucky and Washington D.C. it is almost **EIGHT TIMES**. There is not a single state where it is not at *least* double. These are staggering numbers.

It is reported that over 500,000 black youths are arrested annually for minor marijuana offenses! Now, one can ask: "Why is this so?" Of course one could always argue that the problem is rooted in socio-economics.

I don't see this as relevant in the context of the damage marijuana arrests cause to the future of so many black youths, as well as many white youths as well. Decriminalize first. That's easy. Work on the tough and important socio-economic issues later.

Decriminalization *is* the issue when one considers the billions of dollars spent on law enforcement in apprehending youths for minor marijuana violations. This is on top of the billions of dollars of court costs which follow arrests, and on top of the billions of dollars of incarceration costs thereafter. Could not these billions of dollars be better spent solving the socio-economic problems that are the root cause of most of the marijuana arrests in the first place?

261

Even more important, think of the future earnings potential (and, yes, think of the future income tax potential) that is lost by the "criminal" personal records that follow these kids around for the rest of their lives. Regardless of how well they become educated or how completely some manage to turn around their lives, the stigma of a marijuana conviction follows them for life. It is a stigma that simply never goes away.

It is also sad but true that many, if not most employers will hesitate to hire *anyone* with a criminal record or *any* sort. Possession and/or sale of small amounts of marijuana is one such victimless "crime". Decriminalization of marijuana would open many doors of employment opportunity to many inner-city youths who presently are virtually unemployable because of their arrests for using or selling a harmless herbal medicine.

Because of local laws prohibiting almost all *marijuana industry* companies from hiring anyone with even a minor drug conviction in their past, blacks have been unjustly excluded from participation in this exploding new industry. This was first brought to national attention by the San Francisco NAACP. They are actively backing a black female dispensary license applicant, and are working hard to see more blacks employed in the industry in the future.

We are supposed to be a compassionate country. Here is an absolute no-brainer way to prove it. Decriminalize marijuana possession as so many advanced civilized countries around the world have done (See Appendix IV). Are we neither as civilized nor as advanced nor as compassionate as we like to pretend? I hope that is not the case. Are you listening President Obama? Hillary? Bernie? Anyone?

We have the opportunity in November 2016 to elect a president who can, with the stroke of a pen, decriminalize marijuana possession. Yet in all of the many candidate debates leading up to the election not once has a moderator asked the simple question directly of any candidate: "If elected president would you decriminalize marijuana in the interest of saving countless black youths from a destroyed future?" **Not one. Why do you suppose that is?**

This is not only a simple matter of "legalization". It is not even a matter of reclassification from marijuana's ridiculous Schedule I designation. Those are entirely separate issues dealt with elsewhere in this book. *"Illegal but decriminalized as to possession and sale of small amounts"* is something that no rational, intelligent person can logically argue against.

Arguments against legalization for recreational use may be worthy of some debate. Arguments against legalization for medical use far less so. But arguments against decriminalization in the interest of our youth, both black and white are simply an unconscionable national disgrace.

Marijuana has ruined the lives of more disadvantaged inner-city youths than anything else. This is NOT because of their use of or addiction to marijuana. It is because of needless arrests for possession and/or sale of trivial amounts of *The Wonder Weed*. This not only clogs up the court calendars, but costs taxpayers untold millions of dollars in prison costs. Decriminalization would put this travesty behind us.

WAKE UP AMERICA!

CHAPTER 35
JURY DUTY? WHY SHOULD I CARE?

Whoopie Goldberg, Actress, Academy Award Winner, "The View" Co-Host:
"If you make it legal it becomes like liquor. Like at a liquor store you have to be a certain age to get it, you have to have ID when you go in, you have the different kinds. And it will be utilized and taxed the same way that they do liquor. They'll make money. It's the same that they do with cigarettes."

The Important Connection Between
Marijuana And Jury Duty

It is an unfortunate fact that many individuals make all sorts of excuses to get out of jury duty. It is, in fact, your solemn duty as a free American to see to it that our legal system works as it should. For anyone who is passionate about the legalization of marijuana, you need to go *out of your way* to serve on jury duty. Here's why:

Flashback to the days of alcohol prohibition. Why is alcohol legal today and marijuana illegal? Why was prohibition repealed?

One reason was that the government was desperate, after the Great Depression began in 1929, to raise revenue from somewhere. Alcohol sales were an easy answer. But **why** was it an easy answer?

The fact is, prohibition was an abysmal failure. So is our decades long "War On Drugs" (we *never* learn). The continued illegal status of marijuana will inevitably be known as an equally abysmal failure.

Tax revenue aside, the major reason why prohibition did not work was the difficulty in successfully prosecuting illegal alcohol dealers and users. The key here was **jury trials.** Any defendant demanding a fast jury trial was virtually *certain* to be exonerated. Why? Because, as with marijuana today, a *majority* of the population, *potential jurors all*, favored the end of prohibition!

The odds of selecting a jury where that one vote that would hang the jury was not in the mix was virtually zero! As is the case today with marijuana, the more alcohol jury trials that were scheduled the more clogged the court calendars became. Certain laws governed the right to a jury trial within a certain time limit. It was almost impossible to prosecute *within this time limit.*

So why doesn't every perp almost always plead "guilty"? The reason is "plea bargaining". Faced with possible long jail time and a serious criminal record, many simply choose probation or minimal jail time over possible years of prison. They simply do not want to risk lengthy incarceration.

Is there actually *any* risk in front of a jury in a country where a majority are soft on marijuana and it takes a *single* dissenting vote to hang a jury? You decide. Is this not exactly analogous to alcohol prohibition? I say it is.

The government today actively pursues marijuana dealers and consumers, especially in that majority of unenlightened states that have yet to pass any laws legalizing marijuana, even for medicinal purposes. Selling marijuana is a source of Income in impoverished inner-city areas, perhaps their only possible source.

Because of this a disproportionate number of black youths

suffer prosecution and incarceration. This leads to the lifetime stigma of a criminal record which virtually insures that they can never achieve the American Dream.

If every individual charged with a marijuana "crime" demanded a fast jury trial there would be virtually no black youth convictions! Because of the majority pro-marijuana-legalization sentiment in the United States virtually no jury would *unanimously* vote to convict! At least one (probably more than one) juror would vote "Acquit"!

This exactly parallels what the government learned regarding alcohol prohibition. Why spend untold millions of dollars capturing, temporarily housing, and bringing to trial tens of thousands of individuals with almost no chance to obtain a conviction? As it was with alcohol, legalization of marijuana is a no-brainer.

Prior to prohibition alcohol was a known killer. Thirteen years of prohibition accomplished little positive in the long run. During those years alcohol was readily available on the black market. Criminals got rich. Jury convictions were quite problematic. Elliot Ness and his "Untouchables" were a pimple on an elephant's ass. Tax revenue was being lost.

The government simply gave in to reality. It took far too long for that reality to become the 21st Amendment to the Constitution on December 5, 1933. Legalization of marijuana is an even bigger no-brainer than was the repeal of alcohol prohibition. Marijuana doesn't kill. Alcohol does. It is impossible to "overdose" on marijuana because the active compounds in it do not affect the portion of the brain that controls breathing.

Further, government studies (most of which are poorly

reported if reported at all) have shown that marijuana is NOT a "gateway drug" leading to dangerous addictions.

Most important, marijuana, a simple natural healing herb, has been shown, for thousands of years, to have immensely beneficial curative properties for countless diseases. One component of cannabis, CBD, has been shown to actually cure certain cancers! **Wake up Washington!**

There is an entire new "branch" of legal practice, "Marijuana Specialization". Hundreds of attorneys have jumped on the bandwagon. They are well aware that if they can get their client in front of a jury that acquittal is almost certain.

So, show up for jury duty! Prevent needless and unfair convictions by being the juror-vote that prevents the government from yet another successful marijuana prosecution or life-damaging plea bargain. This is just the sort of cumulative pressure we need to convince the government of the futility of the current marijuana laws.

GOD bless marijuana, GOD bless our court system, and GOD bless America!

CHAPTER 36
<u>WHITE MAN SPEAKS</u>
<u>WITH FORKED TONGUE</u>

<u>Chief Ouray,</u> Utel Tribe, ca 1868:
"An agreement made with the government is like the agreement a buffalo makes with the hunter after it has been pierced by many arrows. All it can do is lie down and give in".

<u>Maia Szalavitz</u>, Neuroscience Journalist, Columnist & Author:
"For the first time ever, a solid majority of Americans supports legalizing marijuana. Some politicians are slowly discovering that lingering fears about being labeled 'soft on crime' for supporting marijuana reform are unwarranted.. While national politicians remain mired in late-'90s thinking that suggests supporting the drug war is the only viable position, national polling trends (especially by age) and state-level political movements indicate that serious consideration of marijuana reform makes sense."

Since winning some of our country from the British, and buying much of it from France, Spain and Russia, we have managed to treat indigenous Americans horribly. I don't feel quite so bad over our stealing Hawaii from Queen Liliuokalani. After all, the Hawaiians themselves forcibly took the Islands from the original Polynesian settlers. What's fair is fair!

Within the continental United States there is a very significant area wherein neither federal nor state laws governing the possession, use, sale or growing marijuana _should_ apply. This is the land designated as Indian Reservations, and it is

268

supposed to be autonomous!

Excluding Alaska, there are about 88,000 square miles (56 million acres) of Indian Reservations in the lower 48 states. There are 43 major recognized tribal groups, and 326 separate recognized tribes (as many as 520 Tribes total).

The approximate population on these reservations is about one million individuals. (Alaska is probably not optimal for growing marijuana, so I'm ignoring it in this Chapter.)

It was *widely* reported in the media in early 2015 that: "ALL INDIAN RESERVATIONS WILL BE ALLOWED TO REGULATE MARIJUANA LAWS!" They apparently could grow all the marijuana they wanted.

This would be the ultimate revenge for the white man appropriating most of the original Tribal Lands. Native Americans could now potentially leave a "Trail of Tears" all the way to the bank! This was the universal and logical understanding of the Department of Justice's initial proclamation. No one doubted the government's sincerity.

Not so fast. It was too good to be true. The Justice Department was at first clearly understood (misunderstood?) to say that it would allow Native American tribes to choose whether or not to legalize marijuana on their reservations, and grow all they wanted to grow.

It seems that under the latest Justice Department regulations, tribes are **_only_** free to **maintain a _ban_** even if the states they are located in have passed medical marijuana laws or even full recreational use laws. ***The opposite is apparently not true***: Tribal efforts at legalization aren't allowed to overrule state laws that criminalize marijuana. Screwed again!

269

So, as in the past, Uncle Sam seems to have spoken with a forked tongue. There are many Tribes that had already begun to try to reap this harvest based on their legitimate understanding of the Justice Department's original edict. Some spent a great deal of money in the process. They are all screwed. This time it's the DOJ, not the US Cavalry. Alexander Hamilton would be proud!

For example, the Pit River Tribe in California spent an enormous amount of money creating a large growing facility. The result: Federal Agents unexpectedly raided their facility and seized 12,000 marijuana plants and a hundred pounds of processed product prepared and ready for sale!

The Menominee tribe in Wisconsin was shocked in October 2015 to have Federal Agents raid *their* growing facility and destroy 30,000 plants! What made this situation somewhat different is the tribe's claims that the plants were industrial hemp designated for research and ***not*** psychoactive marijuana.

Consistent with marijuana and hemp laws on the federal level, as far as the invading Agents were concerned one form of marijuana is just like any other form of marijuana. Idiots.

Wisconsin law is a bit odd in that the state itself enforces criminal violations occurring within the boundaries of most, but not *all*, of Wisconsin's Indian reservations. The Menominee have the *unfortunate* distinction of being the *only* tribe where criminal violations are enforced by federal police agencies and courts. Goodbye 30,000 plants.

Incidentally, growing hemp was illegal in America for decades (an even bigger absurdity than marijuana being illegal) until an amendment to the 2014 Federal Farm Bill *finally* allowed

270

states to at least *begin* to implement pilot hemp programs for "agricultural research".

So what about the ambitious plans of the Idaho Sioux Tribe that had decided to create a marijuana destination *resort*, the first in the USA? They *already* run a successful casino, hotel and buffalo ranch on their reservation. They broke ground for adding a smoking lounge to make their facility a marijuana users' paradise. Are they also screwed? You bet they are! Plans have been abandoned until further notice.

For now Indian Tribes across the country can simply watch as Tribes in Washington and Oregon, with *their* states' very liberal marijuana laws, adhere to their new understanding of federal law. For example, Washington's Squaxin Island Tribe and Squamish Tribe have signed agreements with the state to strictly follow *all* state regulations. The key difference is that tax revenues go to the tribe!

The Confederated Tribes of Warm Springs in Oregon have also proceeded slowly. Like the Squaxin and Squamish Tribes, their approach has been to work hand in hand with all local authorities, rather than to act as independent sovereign Tribes. The feds just *hate* Indian sovereignty.

One Tribe moving forward very cautiously is The Las Vegas Paiute Tribe. They are planning to build an 85,000 square foot grow facility and two dispensaries near the Vegas Strip. They hope to become a model for ALL American Indian Tribes in the future.

General advice from legal authorities to all Indian Tribes: Develop a tight relationship with your State Governor and State Attorney General. Preferably start planning in a state where marijuana is already legal.

Try to build a strong relationship with the US Attorney General (and hope to hell it isn't Chris Christie). The Paiute Tribe model will be watched carefully by tribes nationwide.

For now, in general, Tribal Leaders throughout the United States have come to realize and accept that they cannot grow and sell marijuana on their "autonomous" reservations at this time in most states. They have most certainly not abandoned the idea of entering the extremely lucrative marijuana market as soon as possible. They must simply watch and wait.

The upcoming November 2016 elections are **very** important. This is not just because there may be additional states allowing both medical and recreational use of marijuana, but more so because our next President will be making _two_ very critical appointments.

Both the new Attorney General and the new ninth Supreme Court Justice could have a profound effect on the entire multi-billion-dollar marijuana industry. The very future of marijuana in America, and of course on Indian lands, is at stake.

The marijuana battle lines are being drawn. Ever so slowly sanity is beginning to reign over ignorance, both in the several states and territories, as well as on the Indian reservations. Only time will tell how this will all play out in the future.

CHAPTER 37
POLITICS 2016 AND
HOW TO WIN THE PRESIDENCY

<u>Nancy Pelosi</u>, U.S. House Minority Leader & Former Speaker of the House:
"I have strong concerns about the recent actions by the federal government that threaten the safe access of medicinal marijuana to alleviate the suffering of patients in California...I am pleased to join organizations that support legal access to medicinal marijuana, including the American Nurses Association, the Lymphoma Foundation of America, and the AIDS Action Council."

<u>Jimmy Kimmel</u>, ABC Talk Show Host:
"I do have one real question for you Mr. President, what's with the marijuana crackdown? Mr. President, I hope you don't think I'm out of line here, but marijuana is something that real people care about."

Historically candidates for public office will say pretty much whatever the particular audience to which they are speaking want to hear them say. Marijuana legalization is a very polarizing issue, and it is understandable that taking a firm stand on the issue can gain or lose votes and could even win or lose the presidential election.

For whatever reason, except for a few offhand questions directed at a single candidate, no moderator of any debate, Democrat or Republican, posed the question of legalization directly to any candidate. Yet at one time or another in the past each candidate has made some reference to the topic.

There are critical elections in November 2016. Based on extensive highly-regarded polling data any politician who *openly and without equivocation* declares in favor of decriminalization and legalization of marijuana should win in a landslide over any anti-legalization candidate. The Presidency is no exception. **Are you listening Donald and Hillary? Bernie? IS *ANYONE* OUT THERE LISTENING?**

The following statements are what I have either heard directly on radio and TV, or been able to research. Most of the following individuals are either ex-candidates, potential candidates in the future, or potential members of a newly elected President's cabinet.

We all know that politicians often say one thing and then do another after they are elected. We have studied the present candidates and considered the positions they have taken on medical and recreational marijuana in the past. Based on this, here is my summation as to what we get (and deserve) if we elect, directly or indirectly, one of these individuals.

CLEARLY ANTI-MARIJUANA LEGALIZATION:

New Jersey Governor **Chris Christie** (R) is totally against marijuana for any purpose, medical or recreational. He says he will strongly and immediately strictly enforce existing federal laws. I heard him on TV during an interview say that if elected: "I would see to it that every marijuana dispensary owner is sent to jail!" This misguided totally uninformed clown could actually end up in a key government position.

Christie is quoted as saying: "Residents of the legal-marijuana states better smoke 'em while they got 'em, because as of January 2017, I will enforce the federal laws."

The biggest problem here is that it is a *very real possibility* that in a Trump cabinet Mr. Christie could very well become Attorney General. He also could become the 9th Supreme

Court Justice. If either, GOD forbid, happens, the marijuana legalization movement could be set back decades.

Carly Fiorina (R) is apparently against legalization for either medical or recreational purpose. As the shortest-running vice presidential candidate in history, it is rather unlikely that she will have any significant political influence in the near future.

Mike Huckabee (R) is against legalization for either medical or recreational purposes, I assume on religious grounds.

Jeb Bush (R) is reported to be against legalization for either medical or recreational purposes. He is quoted as saying he would have voted "NO" if he were in a state that was considering legalization. Another idiot.

Rick Santorum (R) is reportedly against legalization for either medical or recreational purposes.

DOCTOR (emphasis intentional) **Ben Carson** (R) sees "*limited value*" for medical marijuana except in "compassionate cases". This essentially mirrors the opinion of Big Pharma. **He surely knows better.** He is also against decriminalization and against the use of recreational marijuana. So is Big Pharma. **Coincidence?** As with Chris Christie, if Dr. Carson ends up in the government, in his case as Surgeon General, legalization is in for a *very* rough ride.

Jim Gilmore (R) has stated a strongly anti-legalization position.

Marco Rubio (R) is against decriminalization and against recreational legalization. For medical use he is only in favor of "non-euphoric" marijuana, which by its narrow definition is essentially anti-medical use. PROBLEM: As with New Jersey Governor Christie he could end up in Mr. Trump's cabinet.

Scott Walker (R) has stated a strongly anti-legalization position.

SOMEWHAT ANTI - LEGALIZATION BUT WITH A MIXED MESSAGE:

Donald Trump (R) our Republican Presidential candidate, is in favor of legalizing medical marijuana, but against decriminalization for recreational use. Known for "evolving positions" on many issues it can only be hoped that he becomes better informed and solidly in favor of full decriminalization and legalization.

If Mr. Trump were to come out in favor of full legalization **before** the election it could help him win in a landslide. But if Ms. Clinton is wise enough to beat him to it, and adopts Bernie Sanders' position, *she* could win the presidency in a landslide!

Bobby Jindal (R) is reported to be in favor of medical marijuana, but against recreational use and against decriminalization.

Lindsay Graham (R) has not made his position totally clear, but appears to support some changes in federal law.

George Pataki (R) has been quoted as having some inclination to changes in federal laws regarding marijuana.

Hillary Clinton (D) is in favor of medical marijuana for "extreme conditions" only. She wants to "wait and see" how things go in the states that have decriminalized and legalized for all medical use and recreational use. She could steamroll Mr. Trump if she declares strongly in favor of unschedulingor rescheduling to Schedule III, and full decriminalization. (See a further discussion of Ms. Clinton below.)

TOPIC - EDUCATED AND WELL INFORMED ABOUT MARIJUANA:

Bernie Sanders (D) is in favor of decriminalization, legalization of medical marijuana, and legalization of recreational marijuana. He is by far the most outspoken of all of the candidates on this issue.

Martin O'Malley (D) is in favor of medical marijuana and decriminalization of small amounts of marijuana. He would reclassify marijuana only as a Schedule II drug. His mind is not made up on recreational marijuana.

Ted Cruz (R) is in favor of States Rights: "Let the states decide both medical and recreational use." This is a good position from the standpoint of decriminalization and legalization.

Rand Paul (R) is in favor of legalization of medical marijuana and in letting the states decide on recreational use. Kentucky Senator Paul has introduced a bill to end the federal ban on medical marijuana! Likewise a good position.

John Kasich (R) Although he previously was in favor of medical legalization only if the FDA gave its approval, he surprisingly signed Ohio Bill 523 into law back in June making Ohio the 25th full medical use state!

Gary Johnson (L) The Libertarian candidate for President is one of the strongest legalization advocates in the USA!

Just in case Ms. Clinton gets indicted for her e-mail indiscretions and/or drops out or goes to jail, I mention three possible replacements:

Joe Biden (D) Vice President Biden has said that he doesn't support criminal actions against marijuana users: "I think the idea of focusing significant resources on interdicting or convicting people for smoking marijuana is a waste of ourresources." "That's different from legalization. Our policy for our Administration is still not legalization, and that is and continues to be our policy."

Al Gore (D) renowned inventor of the internet and valiant savior of polar bears, is a tough call. No record of any position, but generally leans left and supporting marijuana legalization would not be surprising. He has been quoted as saying: "I smoked it in the Army and in college."

Elizabeth Warren (D) "I held my father's hand while he died of cancer, and it's really painful when you do something like that up close and personal... It puts me in a position of saying if there's something a physician can prescribe that can help someone who's suffering, I'm in favor of that. Medical marijuana should be like any other prescription drug. It's really hard to watch someone suffer that you love. My father was sick and there was some conversation about whether or not marijuana would have helped."

Let's talk a bit more about Ms. Clinton. There is a lot more documentation in the media of her various responses when questioned about marijuana legalization than with others.

She says she has never smoked marijuana, not even as an undergraduate in the 1960s. Her husband's administration went nuclear favoring the War on Drugs. During the 2008 campaign, she *publicly opposed marijuana legalization.*

At a 2015 fundraiser in Oregon, a year after that state legalized marijuana, she mentioned working with local officials on "marijuana reform". Everyone present cheered! When questioned afterwards she said: "I am thinking about it. We have to figure out how to thread the needle between the states and the federal government."

Ms. Clinton is also quoted as saying that she wants to "wait and see" how legalization plays out in the states, but has also told a television interviewer that she "doubts the efficacy of medical marijuana." The Clinton campaign declined a donation from the National Cannabis Industry Association according to the NCIA's Executive Director.+

Regarding President Obama's position, she has said: "He has bigger fish to fry than what is happening in Colorado and Washington." Because of this and her other "neutral" statements it is hard to figure exactly how she would stand on decriminalization and legalization if elected President.

The above represents the individuals' positions on marijuana legalization as best I can determine them. As with all issues, any candidate might "reassess" his or her quoted opinions and do a full one-eighty if they perceive some political advantage in so doing in the future.

Rhetorical question: "Does Big Pharma contribute heavily to any of these candidates or their Super- Pacs?" Just wondering…. No, I'm *certain* that they do!

What marijuana industry participants want is **CLARITY**. Could the federal government shut down the entire industry? Yes, it could, however unlikely. Could the federal government get out of the way entirely and allow the states to make all the decisions while sitting back and collecting massive tax revenues? Yes, it could, also somewhat unlikely.

Will the government un-schedule or re-schedule marijuana to Schedule III so that marijuana companies can use federally insured banks? More important doing so would allow marijuana companies to take the same tax deductions as other American companies legally take. Or will the

279

government wimp out and drop marijuana just to Schedule II which will solve absolutely nothing? Time will tell.

Marijuana legalization is the *sleeper* campaign issue out there, and nobody has the guts to say it! The candidates are unlikely to be able to duck the matter for much longer.

LEGALIZATION OF MARIJUANA CAN TRANSCEND POLITICAL AND RELIGIOUS AFFILIATIONS

<u>REPUBLICAN/CONSERVATIVE</u>:

"The amount of money and legal energy being given to prosecute hundreds of thousands of Americans who are caught with a few ounces of marijuana in their jeans simply makes no sense - the kindest way to put it. A sterner way to put it is that it is an outrage, an imposition on basic civil liberties and on the reasonable expenditure of social energy." Author William F. Buckley, Jr., quoted in *The Albuquerque Journal*, June 9, 1993.

<u>DEMOCRAT /LIBERAL:</u>

"Penalties against drug use should not be more damaging to an individual than the use of the drug itself. Nowhere is this more clear than in the laws against the possession of marijuana in private for personal use." Former President Jimmy Carter, in a message to Congress, August 2, **<u>1977.</u>** **NEWS FLASH!! In a brilliant move to win in November the Democratic Platform Committee has <u>finally</u> added a plank promising to review marijuana laws! Republicans had better act favorably or they are DOOMED in 2016.**

<u>RELIGIOUS RIGHT:</u>
"I really believe we should treat marijuana the way we treat

280

beverage alcohol. If people can go into a liquor store and buy a bottle of alcohol and drink it at home legally, then why do we say that the use of this other substance is somehow criminal?"

Pat Robertson, Chairman of the Christian Broadcasting Network, quoted in *The New York Times,* March 7, 2012.

What can *you* do? CONTACT **ALL** OF THE CANDIDATES, or at the very least your favorites. (ANY GOOGLE SEARCH WILL TELL YOU HOW TO REACH ANY OF THEM.)

We firmly believe that *ALL* opposition to legalization derives from **lack of education on the issue**, and from simply believing the years of outright lies that have clouded the chances for legalization for decades. The degree to which Big Pharma and other lobby groups "own" our politicians is clear.

PREDICTION

Because about 90% of Americans favor medical marijuana legalization and over 50% favor full recreational legalization, the first Presidential candidate who publically makes the following statement will sweep into office carrying <u>all fifty states</u>!

"ONE OF MY TOP PRIORITIES AFTER I AM SWORN IN WILL BE TO ISSUE AN EXECUTIVE ORDER REMOVING MARIJUANA FROM THE DRUG SCHEDULE THE SAME AS TOBACCO AND ALCOHOL, DECRIMINALIZING POSSESSION, USE, AND GROWING, AND ALLOWING EVERY STATE AND TERRITORY TO DECIDE ALL ISSUES OF LEGALIZATION WITHOUT ANY FEDERAL INTERVENTION. I WILL ALSO AUTHORIZE THE GROWING OF INDUSTRIAL HEMP NATIONWIDE."

WHY *ISN'T* OUR GOVERNMENT LISTENING? AH, BUT

THEY ARE, APPARENTLY TO THE POWERFUL BIG-PHARMACEUTICAL ANTI-MARIJUANA LOBBY AND THE COMPLICIT, COMPLACENT AND CLUELESS MEDIA. IT IS HARD TO SEE A PATH TO THE WHITE HOUSE FOR ANYCANDIDATE THAT DOES NOT PUT IN SOME SERIOUS THOUGHT AND TIME ON EVERY ASPECT OF THE MARIJUANA LEGALIZATION ISSUE.

WAKE UP AMERICA! HEAR THE CRIERS OF OUR PTSD AFFLICTED VATERANS. HEAR THE CRIES OF CANCER PATIENTS AND MS PATIENTS. HEAR THE CRIES OF CHILDREN WITH SPASTIC DISORDERS. LISTEN CLOSELY. THEN ACT!

TO OUR POLITICIANS I *PLEAD*: "READ THE COUNTLESS SCIENTIFIC REPORTS ON MARIJUANA'S SAFETY AND HEALTH BENEFITS. STUDY THE ISRAELI MEDICAL COMMUNITY'S MARIJUANA/CANCER RESEARCH. **READ *THIS* BOOK THOROUGHLY.**"

THEN MAKE EDUCATED DECISIONS ON FULL LEGALIZATION AND RECLASSIFICATION. SHOW SOME REAL HUMANITY. SHOW SOME REAL BACKBONE. UNCLASSIFY OR RECLASSIFY TO SCHEDULE III, DECRIMINALIZE, AND LEGALIZE MARIJUANA NOW!

If you want to help and participate in our cause, please go to our informative website and sign up for our free newsletter. If you wish to support our cause in any way possible you can donate any amount on our extremely secure encrypted website at: TNWLF.org (The National Weed Legalization Fund).

Thanks!

CHAPTER 38
COMPASSIONATE ACTIONS
YOU CAN TAKE NOW

Ann Landers, Advice Columnist:
I have long believed the laws regarding marijuana are too harsh. Those who keep pot for their own personal use should not be treated as criminals. Thirty years in prison makes no sense whatsoever."

HELP US LEGALIZE MARIJUANA! Call it cannabis, weed, pot, ganja, MaryJane or grass there is absolutely **no good logical reason** for possession , and medical and recreational use of GOD's natural healing herbal plant **to be illegal**.

Massive amounts of documentation dating back thousands of years offers conclusive proof of the medicinal value of marijuana for many very serious ailments for countless patients. Recreationally, let's compare annual deaths: from tobacco (450,000); from alcohol (30,000); from prescription drugs (20,000); and from cocaine, heroin, bath salts, ecstasy and similar illegal drugs (100,000 estimated.) **Deaths from marijuana use: ZERO! Duh. Double duh!**

Current ineffective restrictive laws do not even begin to prevent the widespread availability and use of street-marijuana anywhere in the United States. Plans to reclassify marijuana down to a Schedule II drug are a meaningless distraction. It MUST be either un-scheduled along with tobacco and alcohol, or moved to Schedule III or higher.

Planned federal studies of one single "pure" strain (there are thousands of strains, each with a unique chemistry and use) are an equally meaningless waste of time and resources, and an obvious tactic to delay legalization indefinitely.

Together we can:

- Free up the overburdened court system;
- Raise many billions in new federal, state and local tax revenues;
- Stop incarcerating black teens and ruining their chances in life;
- Save many billions in jail costs;
- Create millions of new jobs nationwide!

Which of these goals is worthy of *any* opposition?
I cannot think of one. Can you?

PREDICTION: ANY political candidate for President who has the nerve and will to promise rapid de-classification, reclassification and FULL LEGALIZATION by Executive Order if elected will win in a landslide! Will any have the guts to do so? We shall see.

No other issue is more real and personally-important to a polled majority of Americans of every political persuasion than decriminalization and legalization of marijuana. Almost 90% favor medical marijuana, and over 50% favor full recreational use. The time for action is NOW! Alaska, Colorado, D.C., Oregon and Washington got it right!

The National Weed Legalization Fund is an Arizona non-profit corporation. We are a fledgling company and need your help to raise significant funds for radio and TV ads, magazine ads, political lobbying, celebrity lobbying, mailings, surveys and a periodic newsletter. Any and all donations of any amount will be appreciated. Do your part. Spread the word through ALL of your social media contacts. Please check out our website at: thenationalweedlegalizationfund.org **AND DONATE NOW!**

There are MANY fine non-profit groups who do fantastic lobbying for marijuana legalization. Collectively they are the reason we are making progress. Please see Appendix II, check out their websites, and consider donating on these sites as well.

Write to your two Senators. Write to your Representatives. Write to your Governor. Write to your Mayor. Below is a suggested letter to government officials. Please consider using it, or create something similar. Thank you in advance for your kind and generous support.

SUGGESTED LETTER TO GOVERNMENT OFFICIALS

Dear xxxxxxxxxxxxxxxxxxxxxxxxxxx:

We desperately need your help.

As you know, the War On Drugs has been an abysmal failure. Just as with alcohol during prohibition in the 1920s, making possession and use of marijuana illegal has not prevented the cartels from providing easy access to marijuana everywhere.

Together we can:

- Free up the overburdened court system;
- Raise many billions in new Federal, State and local tax revenues;
- Stop incarcerating poor black teens and ruining their

chances in life;
- Save many millions in police and jail costs;
- Create millions of new jobs.

Which of these achievable goals is worthy of your opposition? I cannot think of one.

No other issue is more real and personally-important to a polled majority of Americans of every age and political persuasion than legalization of marijuana. Around 90% favor medical marijuana, and over 50% favor full recreational use. The time for action is NOW. Five venues got it right!

Marijuana *must* be federally rescheduled. It does not belong categorized alongside heroin and crack-cocaine in Schedule I. It should be un-scheduled, as with deadly tobacco and alcohol. It could be upgraded to at least a Schedule III drug.

Marijuana has been shown conclusively to be a powerful and very safe medicine. It is proven effective for a wide range of ailments. **It should be taxed and regulated the same as alcohol and tobacco.**

Although fully legal, alcohol and tobacco kill hundreds of thousands of Americans every year. Marijuana has NEVER killed anyone! It cannot kill at any dose. It is not just the thousands of years of anecdotal evidence that has shown all of this to be true.

There have been thousands of scientific studies, including our own government's studies going back to New York City Mayor Fiorello La Guardia and President Richard Nixon, that pleaded for legalization.

It is very important to understand WHY marijuana is considered illegal. It was a conspiracy between media mogul

William Randolph Hearst and Harry Anslinger that created the "marihuana" absurd terror campaign in the mid-1930s.

Anslinger needed a job after alcohol prohibition failed. Hearst needed to protect his timber and paper businesses. They made a powerful team. Their evil conspiracy has prevented hundreds of millions of Americans from obtaining blessed relief from pain and suffering for decades. It has destroyed the lives of millions of black youths.

It has contributed to the *loss* of **millions of American lives** to the ravages of alcohol , tobacco, and opiate drugs, all of which marijuana can replace to a greater or lesser extent.

Anslinger and Hearst made up total lies, used only the term "marihuana", and fear of "evil" Mexicans, in lieu of "cannabis". Cannabis was a familiar term to all Americans. It had been a major constituent in dozens of popular medicines since the late 1890s.

Sadly there are **huge** lobby interests at play in this matter. Big Pharma stands to lose millions of dollars from lost opioid pain killer revenue, and the profits from other deadly prescription drugs. Big Timber is terrified of hemp farming, a harmless form of marijuana that could replace the high-pollution tree-based paper industry. Big Tobacco and Big Alcohol could also stand to lose, as could Big Private Prisons.

The amount of lobby-money and perks these mega-corporations bring to the table to influence our politicians and the media is enormous. It is clear to anyone that these powerful lobbies are the **primary** influence for the long-standing opposition to legalization by most doctors and many if not most politicians.

Please (insert name of official), take the time to learn the real truth about marijuana. There are many excellent informative books in print, including the recently-published *"MARIJUANA – THE WONDER WEED"*.

Please listen to the voices of your constituents. Do everything in your power to promote legalization of this wonderful natural GOD-given herbal medicine.

Thank you for your kind attention to this letter.

Sincerely,

(Be sure to sign each letter individually.)

THE MORE OF THESE LETTERS YOU CAN SEND OUT THE BETTER!

If you want to help and participate in our cause, please go to our informative website and sign up for our free newsletter. If you wish to support our cause in any way possible you can donate any amount on our extremely secure encrypted website at: TNWLF.org (The National Weed Legalization Fund).

Thanks!

CHAPTER 39
FINAL THOUGHTS

Dean Becker, **Syndicated Radio Host & Former USAF Security Policeman:**
"In the name of all the powers that be, let us reconsider our stance regarding the policy of drug prohibition. In this hundred year effort to prevent the use of certain flowers and plant extracts we have empowered criminal elements worldwide to the tune of $400 billion per year. The US has arrested 39 million non-violent drug users at a cost of more than one trillion dollars."

I hope that you have read this book carefully. Forgive me if some Chapters were a bit too technical. As a chemical engineer I have a genetic predisposition for writing out long chemical names!

I also apologize if I took the liberty of repeating certain events and certain arguments in more than one Chapter. My purpose was to emphasize a few key points that were pivotal in the long battle for marijuana legalization.

Legalization of marijuana for medical purposes is such a no-brainer that it is difficult to make any hard valid argument against it. Recreational use could bring in massive tax revenue, and create millions of jobs, and cause little harm.

As a side benefit it might just relax our overwound-spring of a society and in general create some level of peace and serenity. Marijuana is a very powerful relaxant.

Decriminalization of possession is perhaps the greatest no-brainer of all. The damage that has already been done to millions of our precious youth, especially inner city blacks, is a national disgrace.

The money that could be saved by eliminating the incarcerations alone could be in the billions of dollars! Decriminalization offers the added benefit of freeing up the police for pursuing the more pressing felonious crimes.

We teeter on a very precarious edge somewhere between total federal criminalization nationwide and total state's rights to decide every legalization issue. For the moment at least the government has taken a "hands off" "states' rights" approach. Unfortunately that could change in a heartbeat .....or a pen-stroke.

It could literally change overnight depending on the politics of the next President. At least one former Republican candidate, and possible future Attorney General, has pledged to put all legal medical marijuana dispensary owners in prison the day after he is elected! In totally the opposite approach Democrat (Socialist?) Bernie Sanders has pledged full legalization if he is elected! Go Bernie!

A major potential problem the industry as a whole faces is the ever-present possibility of changes in *local* laws that shut down dispensaries and grow operations that were *initially ruled **legal**.* Cases in point, Montana, and Vancouver, Canada as discussed in Appendices later in this book.

Of course the federally-illegal status has caused incredible hardship in the industry. It is impossible for a legal marijuana business to open a bank account to deposit its funds. Come tax time marijuana-related business expenses may not be tax-deductible. Taxes must be paid on *gross* sales, which makes turning a profit virtually impossible for some companies. This is especially true in an industry that is very heavily regulated seed to sale. Worse, should a marijuana business find itself in financial trouble, they cannot file for any federal Bankruptcy Chapter protection. Ouch!

The thousands of years of evidence in favor of marijuana is overwhelming. Allowing tobacco and alcohol to be freely bought in any quantity, and not allowing marijuana's medical and recreational use is literally criminal.

The key to full legalization both medical *and* recreational is **_public education._** Educational advocacy groups (See Appendix II) such as The *National Organization for the Reform of Marijuana Laws* (NORML) and my Arizona non-profit: *The National Weed Legalization Fund* (TNWLF.org) need all the funding they can get to spread the truth where it can best be served. **Please help if you can.**

There are 5,000 years of history of positive marijuana use to draw upon. There are hundreds of real peer-reviewed scientific studies that overwhelmingly support the premise that marijuana is a safe, non-gateway, herbal medicine, not a dangerous addictive Devil- drug.

Many of these are actually <u>federal government funded studies</u> going back to the FDR era. The results were invariably suppressed because they never supported the federal anti-marijuana premise that they were intended in the first place to prove!

The fact is, going back to the '30s ridiculous movie "*Reefer Madness*", there has been a concerted effort to produce total lies and egregious misinformation about marijuana. This has been so constant and pervasive , continuing to this very day, that much of the American public accepts the "evils of marijuana" as most likely being absolutely factual.

In Chapter 5 I mentioned that there were eight social factors I believed decriminalization and legalization of marijuana would reduce. I hope the information presented in this book has offered some level of verification of these contentions:

- *Unemployment and underemployment.* The marijuana industry has proven in Colorado, Oregon and other venues that already have legalization that many thousands of *new* jobs are created and tax revenue skyrockets. <u>These are jobs that *never* before existed.</u>

- *Poverty and racial unrest:* The incarceration of hundreds of thousands of black youths, and the negative employment consequences of a criminal record must be ended. When it is it can only go a long way to reducing black unemployment and the racial unrest that accompanies it.

- *Addiction to alcohol and tobacco.* Marijuana use is a far safer alternative to addictive alcohol and tobacco use. Regular use will reduce both addictions over time.

- *Chronic obesity.* Properly applied medical marijuana can be effectively used in a weight loss regimen. Use has been shown to reduce Body Mass Index (BMI).

- *Prescription drug addiction.* We have an opioid **epidemic** in the United States. Marijuana is a proven pain killer and a definite safe replacement for opioids, especially for PTSD afflicted veterans.

- *Street drug addiction.* Ready availability of quality marijuana is a safe alternative to deadly street drugs and could save thousands of young lives.

- *Severe illnesses, cancer, HIV, and dozens more.* The evidence, both anecdotal and scientifically researched, is overwhelming!

I sincerely hope that the information in this book will lead some to think twice about their opposition to marijuana.

Marijuana is proven to greatly help our PTSD veterans and can help reduce the twenty-two or more DAILY veteran suicides. Yet the VA was until recently prohibited from prescribing it. It is proven to help cancer patients endure chemotherapy. It is proven to help multiple sclerosis patients and other neuro-degenerative disease patients lead a normal life. It is a proven reliever of chronic pain.

An on-going scientific study in Israel is even showing that it has the real potential to actually CURE some cancers. Yet our federal government turns its back on reality and allows our citizens to suffer and die needlessly year after year after year.

Sadly, no one thinks twice about the known dangers of legal cigarette smoking and legal alcohol consumption which have led to literally *millions* of deaths. Marijuana leads to none. How can our government in good conscience turn their backs on the truth? Very, very sad.

Marijuana should be removed entirely from federal drug Scheduling, exactly the same as tobacco and alcohol. Everyone knows that cigarettes kill hundreds of thousands. Do you have any doubts about the dangers of alcohol? Professor David Nutt, a Director at the Division of Brain Sciences at Imperial College in London recently polled a panel of addiction experts.

The professor wanted to know their opinion consensus on the three most dangerous drugs worldwide, based on a number of criteria. They considered dozens of candidate drugs. The result: Heroin is the worst. Cocaine was #3. The consensus for the #2 most dangerous drug: **ALCOHOL!** Point made.

Education aside, the one single impetus for universal legalization is TAX REVENUE. It's not necessarily the morally correct reason, but it is a fact.

In these difficult economic times with the government carrying an unimaginable twenty <u>trillion</u> dollars in funded debt (and five times that in overall debt.....truly incomprehensible numbers) and the states scrambling for funds to cover entitlement programs and unfunded pensions, the potential for this new revenue stream is almost beyond temptation!

The battle to allow full federal legalization of marijuana for any purpose is VERY slowly being won. Perhaps by the time you read this book more of the battle WILL be won. The medical-use battle, at least on the state level, is accelerating steadily. We must first win the legalization war in EVERY state. We must elect a President who has the patience to actually study and learn the facts about marijuana and not succumb to the many deep-pocket anti-marijuana lobbies.

As pointed out in an earlier Chapter, with thousands of strains, and hundreds of cannabinoids and terpenes and their various oxidation products, and various ways to use the products, it is abundantly clear that true scientific research cannot possibly be applied to every possible iteration of these variables in our lifetime.

It would take a hundred years or more of massive research efforts to even scratch the surface of possible research projects. This is why ***ANECTDOTAL EVIDENCE*** plus already *existing* published scientific studies is the **ONLY** logical fast way for those who suffer from a variety of ailments to ever come *close* to finding the ideal strain and delivery method for their particular medical or recreational need.

A potential new force was created recently by Jocelyn Elders, the former United States Surgeon General. She has recruited over _fifty_ very prominent physicians and key medical school professors. This very credible group will be lobbying hard for marijuana legalization. They call the group: "Doctors for Cannabis Regulation". We wish them well.

In a rather surprising move the USFDA has granted GW Pharmaceuticals of England the OK to conduct tests in the United States of their newest CBD-based marijuana product "Epidiolex". These tests will be limited to three rare forms of epilepsy: Dravet Syndrome; Lennox-Gastaut Syndrome; and Tuberous Sclerosis Complex.

The FDA gives a special "orphan drug" designation as incentives for studies of the effects of marijuana on rare diseases with under 200,000 sufferers. GW Pharma has somehow _also_ been given the green light to study their Sativex Spray, intended for MS patients, in the United States.

An important major force pushing for legalization is the labor unions. They are salivating over the huge potential for new members based on new jobs to be created in the marijuana growing and medibles areas in particular.

The United Food and Commercial Workers Union (1.3 million members) has a program called: "Cannabis Workers Rising". They are making inroads in Hawaii, California, Colorado, Oregon, New York and New Jersey in particular.

IS MARIJUANA FINALLY GOING MAINSTREAM?

Walgreen's Pharmacy, a major national chain, has become one of the first "household name" companies to address the matter of medical marijuana in _any_ way. A recent post on Walgreens' "Stay Well" Tumblr blog states: "Research has also shown marijuana provides pain relief in ways that traditional medicines don't. Medical marijuana can improve appetite and relieve nausea in those undergoing cancer chemotherapy, and may even relieve symptoms." **This is incredible stuff coming from a major pharmacy!**

Don't let Big Pharma win this war! Don't let them influence our elected officials through lobbying and donations. **Marijuana should immediately be decriminalized, un-classified (as with alcohol and tobacco) or re-classified to at least Schedule III, regulated and taxed, left up to the states, and made universally available for any purpose.**

American laws are archaic and tragically out of touch. The American Medical Association's (AMA's) own official position since 2009 is stated as: "Marijuana reduces neuropathic pain, and may relieve spasticity and pain in patients with multiple sclerosis. The Schedule I status of marijuana should be reviewed with the goal of facilitating clinical research and development of cannabinoid based medicines and alternative delivery methods." *That was stated seven years ago!*

Of course, this AMA position clearly favors only a Schedule II "clinical research" reclassification which would be a disaster as previously discussed above.

Look closely at the irrefutable evidence that marijuana can dramatically help veterans with PTSD. Understand that it can get veterans off powerful poisonous cocktails of opioids and anti-depressants prescribed by the VA. It could possibly prevent many, if not most, of the twenty-two-plus *daily* veteran suicides.

Forgetting all else, just on behalf of our veterans, anyone with half a brain and any level of compassion should recognize that the government 's stubborn insistence on federal Schedule I for marijuana is an **outrageous national disgrace.**

Polls show that the majority of Americans, perhaps 90%, have been convinced that medical-use marijuana makes great sense and should be legalized nationally. Medical marijuana is becoming an unstoppable political force. Unfortunately the anti-marijuana lobby and the federal government still have almost half the public hesitant over *recreational* use due to decades of lies and gross inflammatory anti-marijuana misinformation

Our society must demand an end to the prohibition of this wonderful healing herbal plant for any and all purposes!

For all of those who have profited for decades off of the misery and suffering of the sick and dying by perpetuating the outright lie that marijuana should be a Schedule I drug that has no redeeming medicinal qualities I say: "You and your Boards of Directors and your investors should be swiftly and permanently dismantled and sent straight away to the dung heap of history."

As I write this, the federal Drug Enforcement Agency (DEA) is said to be "considering" rescheduling marijuana. The key point is, to which Schedule will they go? Moving it to Schedule II would be an almost meaningless gesture. In fact, Schedule IIs endless "scientific one-strain studies" with no benefits whatsoever to the present industry would be a travesty. By the time you are reading this we may know the result.

Un-scheduling or rescheduling marijuana and its derivative products to Schedule III or higher , decriminalizing possession, and treating it the same as alcohol and tobacco would be the single greatest boon possible to the entire marijuana industry.

Over a dozen states' legislatures are in the process of creating bills for voters to pass or kill this coming November

2016. Some bills promote only medicinal use. Some are for full legalization including recreational use. In many states where medicinal use is already approved, there is a push for full recreational use.

The stifling bureaucracy within our government is perhaps the biggest barrier to progress on marijuana legislation. Earlier I outlined three federal authorities that must approve any drug trial: The Drug Enforcement Agency (DEA), The Department of Health (DOH), and The Food and Drug Administration (FDA). They do not work simultaneously, but sequentially.

I only recently became acutely aware of the fact that there are various committees within both Houses of Congress that *also* need to debate and pass on this sort of legalization before it even *gets to* the above Agencies! As I write this the House of Representatives is beating to death the "Comprehensive Addiction and Reform Act". This is in recognition of the opioid addiction epidemic in America.

The solution to the opioid epidemic proposed to be funded through this bill? Marijuana legalization? Of course not! **Opioid reversal drugs!**   Here is yet another example of Big Pharma creating an horrendous problem and then creating yet another drug to fix it! What a business model! How about "The Comprehensive *Marijuana* Reform Act"? Don't hold your breath waiting for *that* bill.

Wake up America! Support *any* political candidate who has the guts to publically support legalization. Consider the evidence beyond PTSD, evidence that includes cancer, ALS, AIDS, multiple sclerosis and a host of other diseases among the maladies relieved or possibly even cured by marijuana.

No civilized society should allow millions of its citizens to suffer needlessly because of corporate greed and media sensationalism.   Please read this book thoroughly. Surf the internet. Study the irrefutable evidence. **Learn the truth**, and vote accordingly.

Here is an amazing statistic: **It is a fact that about ninety percent (90%) of the United States population presently resides in a state that has at least *some* medical marijuana legislation on the books! I have never seen this figure published anywhere else! (See Appendix III for details.)**

Obviously there has been **tremendous** progress at the *state* level over the past decade (damn little at the *federal* level). But only a scant <u>eight percent</u> (8%) of Americans live in those few enlightened venues where *recreational* marijuana is permitted. Only about fifty percent (53%), half of all Americans, live in states with comprehensive medical marijuana laws. **We still have a long way to go.**

The President has unilaterally decided that it is OK for a grown "man" to take a whizz in a bathroom with a young girl, teen or grown woman present. This seems to be an *open invitation* to rapists and pedophiles.

It would appear to me to be far easier, less earth-shocking, and do a hell of a lot more good for the vast majority of our citizens for the President to decriminalize and un-Schedule marijuana with the same simple stroke of his pen.

I leave you with one last thought. Remember my "First News" discussion earlier? Well, I am beginning to see a very disturbing trend in current crime reporting. On a few occasions recently the reporter added: <u>"It is suspected that marijuana use was involved".</u> Suspected by whom, the corrupt reporter? His editor? Big Pharma? Pure bullshit.

One recent article was almost identical to the 1940s "child ax murder" false reporting. Some guy beat up his girlfriend in what was described in the report as a "marijuana induced rage". Really? I have never seen one single anecdotal report or study that ever even *suggested* that marijuana induces any violence in a user. <u>Marijuana's effect is exactly the opposite! It calms users down! The media lies will never cease.</u>

As we get closer to decriminalization and legalization you will see more and more of this sort of corrupt reporting. This goes back to the Hearst/Anslinger total lies of the '30s. Do not think for a moment that big lobby dollars do not directly influence the media. They always have and always will.

Follow the November 2016 election results closely. Florida, Missouri and Oklahoma may go full medical use. Nevada, Maine, California, Arizona, North Dakota, Massachusetts, and Montana and could join the recreational ranks. We can only hope, pray, and lobby!

Screw the greedy drug companies who turn out killer opioids and anti-depressants by the billions. Don't allow their bottomless treasure chests to continue to allow our citizens, and especially our brave veterans, to suffer and die.

<u>DECRIMINALIZE AND LEGALIZE MARIJUANA NOW!</u>

THANK YOU SINCERELY FOR BUYING AND READING THIS BOOK!

If you have any comments or suggestions, please send them to us at: Lions Pride Publishing, PO Box 2100, Green Valley, Arizona 85622.

We would also be very appreciative if you would send us a brief review of you opinion of the book.

You can also contact us by email at: **burta193811@yahoo.com.**

Also, if you would like to help us in our lobbying efforts, please donate any amount, small or large, to our Arizona non-profit organization: The National Weed Legalization Fund at: TNWLF.org.

The website is fully encrypted http<u>s</u>, and we NEVER sell or share any information you choose to give us.

ABOUT THE AUTHOR

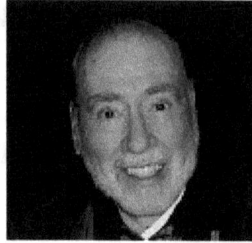

James Burton "Burt" Anderson was born in Brooklyn, New York, where he attended Erasmus Hall High School and the Brooklyn Polytechnic Institute. After earning his degree in Chemical Engineering, he earned his MBA in Management at The Baruch Business College of CCNY. Both degrees were earned in night school over ten years while Burt worked demanding 9 to 5 jobs! He was elected to MuGammaTau, the National Management Honor Society.

For much of his corporate career Burt held high management positions in Fortune 500 Divisions, and served on many Boards of Directors. Recently he was Chief Operating Officer and Board Secretary for Judicate, The National Private Court System. Over the years he has won many impressive sales achievement awards.

As an entrepreneur he has held licenses as a General Securities Principal, Municipal Securities Principal, Real Estate Broker, Financial Advisor, Insurance Broker and Mortgage Broker. He has been a Notary Public in various states. At present he owns Burt Anderson Real Estate in Arizona. He is a Registered Financial Planner.

Burt is an accomplished public speaker and sales trainer,

having shared the podium with the likes of Art Linkletter and Tom Hopkins. He has hosted his own Tucson cable TV talk show, and was featured in a thirty minute infomercial filmed at CBS-Orlando studios with world-famous internet guru Anthony Morrison.

During a brief religious period, Burt became an ordained and licensed Christian minister.

Always interested in giving back to his community, he has served on the Boards of Directors for a number of local non-profit groups. He is an active Chamber of Commerce Member. Burt served for a number of years as the Education Chairman for the Kona-Kohala Board of Realtors in Hawaii.

An author since 1970, he has written over thirty books and countless articles. He was honored to be invited to write an article for *Leaders Magazine* which is distributed only to Heads of State and CEOs.

Burt is an Army veteran, and active member of The American Legion Post #66 in Green Valley, Arizona. Having resided in both Australia and England, and travelled to over thirty countries and every state, he has accumulated a deep understanding of other cultures. His eclectic mix of books draw upon this experience.

Stricken with relapsing/remitting multiple sclerosis in the '70s he has been able to fully control his worst symptoms through the use of marijuana derivatives. For this and other reasons he became extremely active as an advocate for the legalization of medical marijuana.

He is most proud of his achievements as a golfer! He is the only two-time winner of the Burns and Roe Long Island Open, and gold medal winner recently in the local Senior Olympics golf tournament. He also won his college's first Alumni Championship! A lover of competition, he has won 37 Senior Olympics medals over the past decade in golf, pistol and rifle, billiards and basketball! Not half bad for a guy with MS!

Burt is a private pilot, and certified SCUBA diver. After 50+ years of membership he is one of the surviving original members of American MENSA. (His IQ is off the charts!) In 2015 he founded the Arizona non-profit corporation "The National Weed Legalization Fund".   He is currently an engineering consultant and blog writer for a new Tucson multi-divisional marijuana company.

After spending six years reading every related book and scientific study he could access, Burt decided to drop all else and spend a year writing *Marijuana – The Wonder Weed*. He did this in the hope of providing enough information to his readers so that those who may not be well informed might come to a reasoned conclusion in favor of legalization and vote accordingly.

In his 79th year Burt shows few signs of slowing down. He continues to live up to his childhood nickname "RM", which stood for "Renaissance Man"!

He has been married for 33 years to his much younger wife Melanie. They share their home in the High Sonoran Desert with a wonderful dog named Gracie and a cute new (rather destructive!) puppy named Piper.

Melanie, a Vanderbilt grad and ex special-education teacher, has a 9 to 5 job in real estate, yet manages to find the time to tend to their acres of gardens and over 251 household plants! The furthest thing from either of their minds is retirement!

SOME IN-PRINT BOOKS BY THE AUTHOR
AVAILABLE ON AMAZON, KINDLE AND SMASHWORDS

1. *Money By Internet, Volumes I & II.* Over 1,000 pages combined! Proven ways to make money from home sitting in your pajamas in front of a computer screen! The author has been an active infopreneur and internet affiliate-marketer for over two decades.

2. *The Black Belt.* Edited. From the personal notes of a well-known 7th Degree Black Belt karateka, this book provides the average person with easy techniques for easy every-day self-protection.

3. *How To Self-Publish.* From the author's personal success with his company since 1970, Lions Pride Publishing. Write now, publish today!

4. *Reverse Mortgage Dangers.* Valuable information for seniors based upon years of the author's personal experiences as a Loan Officer specializing in Reverse Mortgages. Beware this dangerous product!

5. *Reverse Mortgage Risks.* An expanded and updated sequel to 4.

6. *Making Money From Domain Names.* The author has invested in, and profited from, internet domain names and internet commerce since the mid-'90s. He continues to be involved actively to this day.

7. *Apocalypse 12-21-12 The Mayan Prophesies.* A scholarly work that is not as outdated as the title might imply.

SEVEN BOOKS FROM THE AUTHOR
AVAILABLE LATER IN 2016

1. *The Wit and Wisdom of the Tajiks.* Edited: Translations and interpretations of proverbs from a Christian missionary living in Tajikistan.

2. *Digger The Cat.* Illustrated by (FIVERR.com). An interactive adventure/mystery story for children. (Also to be available in a CD version.)

3. *A Miner's Tailings.* The commissioned biography of an old-time Arizona gold miner and WWII Atom-Bomb aviator. Incredible surprising story!

4. *Martial Arts Trailblazer.* The only authorized biography of Great Grand Master Aaron Banks, the legendary father of mixed martial arts in America. Among his students and fascinating stories: Muhammad Ali, Joe Namath, Marilyn Monroe, Chuck Norris, Buddy Rich, 007 Roger Moore, Bruce Lee, and dozens more!

5. *Astrology and Your Pet.* If you believe in human astrology, you'll be fascinated to learn that your pet is similarly influenced. Amazing!

6. *Mongol Recipes – Genghis Kahn's Cuisine.* The first in an anticipated series of twenty or more unique ethnic cookbooks.

7. *How To Win At Golf – The Easy Way!* A lighthearted look at golf as it is played at the sub-amateur hacker's level. Mulligans galore!

APPENDIX I
THE MARIJUANA DICTIONARY

Every separate discipline has its share of slang terms. Teenagers have a language all their own. Social media has given rise to countless words that were not seen in any dictionary a decade ago.

Every industry...steel, oil, textiles...you name it, has a "slang" language understood best by those who participate daily. The realm of marijuana over the centuries seems to have produced more slang terms than any other area of human endeavor!

The following is a far from complete dictionary of terms that are familiar to most serious marijuana users:

4:20 (420, 4/20):   A commonly used slang term for "smoking marijuana", or "it's time to smoke". It apparently originated at San Rafael High School in California in the early '70s where students coined the phrase to communicate: "4:20PM - It's time to get high!" April 20th (4/20) is often celebrated with marijuana parties nationwide. It is National Marijuana Day!

Acapulco Gold: A vintage '60s marijuana strain from Acapulco, Mexico.

acid: Slang for the hallucinogen LSD.

adulteration: The finished marijuana herbal product can be sprayed with sugar solution or salt solution to enhance the taste of a low quality bud. More important, it adds to the weight thereby adding to the seller's profits. Adding inexpensive ground oregano, identical in appearance to ground marijuana, is also a common adulterant.

alcohol: A legal intoxicant since the end of prohibition, not federally classified as a drug. It is well documented that it kills thousands of individuals yearly. (My mother died of alcohol induced liver cirrhosis in her 40s.)   Many strongly believe that legalizing marijuana will greatly reduce alcohol consumption and accordingly reduce alcohol-related deaths.

Amsterdam: A city in The Netherlands, Europe. It draws around five million tourists every year, mostly because of marijuana. It is considered a "soft drug" and everything, including recreational use AND growing, is tolerated for "personal use". It is the legal "coffee shops" that draw the tourists.

Anslinger, Harry J.: The primary reason why marijuana is illegal in the United States today is the fact that this evil bastard needed a job after prohibition was repealed!

apple bong: A bong created by strategically drilling three holes in an apple.

aqualung: Slang for a gravity bong.

Aunt Mary: Slang term for marijuana.

Ayurvedic: A traditional Asian Indian medical system, originating over 3,000 years ago. Marijuana is a key part.

bag: The most common way to package an ounce or less of marijuana is in a small zip-lock bag.

bag seed: Common term for seed of unknown origin found in a bag of marijuana.

baked: Feeling of complete intoxication.

bat: Slang for a "one hitter".

Bath Salts: A generic term for a wide variety of extremely

dangerous synthetic street drugs, causing long-term and permanent physical harm. They are variants of the chemical cathinone.

BC: British Columbia, Canada. Vancouver is the stoner capital of North America, with an estimated 20,000 illegal growers!

beans: Marijuana seeds.

beasters: American term for mid-grade Canadian marijuana.

bhang: Asian Indian term for marijuana.

bhang lassi: Popular Asian Indian drink made of marijuana, yoghurt or fermented milk, spices and ice water. Sold in some government-sponsored stores.

BHO: Butane Hash Oils. These are concentrates made by a dangerous process called "butane extraction". They often contain butane residue as a contaminant.

binger: Slang for a bong hit.

blasted: Feeling of complete intoxication.

blazed: Feeling of complete intoxication.

BLD: "Broad Leaf Drug". The cannabis Indica strain.

blowback: The possible result of a "shotgun".

blunt: A marijuana cigarette rolled in a hollowed empty cigar wrapper.

Bogarting a joint: Taking more than two puffs before passing, preferably always to the left. Named after Humphrey Bogart.

boo: Slang term for marijuana.

bomb: "The Bomb" is the best grade marijuana available at the moment.

bone: Street slang for a joint. "Let's smoke a bone dude."

bong: The name is derived from the Thai word "baung" which in Thailand is a crude device made from a hollow bamboo tube. Bongs are next step up from the simple bowl. A commercial bong is a fascinating glass contraption that could grace any chemical lab! It consists of a vertical pipe-like bowl with a closed base so that it can hold water. Then there are two small "straws", one larger than the other (the female straw) and the smaller (male) straw (with the bowl on one end) inserted in it.

bowl: The stoner's specialty accessory glassware. They come is a vast variety of colors, shapes and decoration. In fact, any waterproof container will do. You add a straw with a hole below the water, a second hole (the carburetor) above the water, and a mouthpiece for inhaling (you don't actually need a mouthpiece). It is essentially a poor-man's bong.

brick: A large quantity of low grade marijuana, often a kilogram, pressed into a brick-shaped block. Often glued together with CocaCola.

brownies: Edible marijuana product, easily created using store-bought brownie mix and bud butter.

bubble hash: Cannabis glands extracted using a cold water process.

bubble roll: See "Mendocino Cigar".

bud butter: This is the staple used in most marijuana-edibles recipes. It is easily made on the kitchen stove melting butter with marijuana. There are various recipes for creating it available in any marijuana cookbook. Once made it is stored in the refrigerator just as Land Of Lakes!

buddah: Hip-hop slang for marijuana.

bunk bud: Low quality marijuana.

burnt: Feeling of complete intoxication.

butane hash oil: Concentrates made by a process known as butane extraction.

cabbage: British slang for low grade marijuana (schwag).

caned: British slang equivalent to American "stoned".

cannabidiol (CBD): The second most common cannabinoid found in marijuana. It is the non-intoxicating cannabinoid which does not attach to the brain's CB1 receptor, but only to the CB2 receptors outside the brain. It is known to relieve convulsions, inflammation, anxiety, nausea, and inhibit cancer cell growth.

cannabinoids: A class of chemical molecules produced by all marijuana plants in varying quantities. Many of these react with the human nervous system with a wide variety of effects.

cannabis: The botanical genus name for marijuana and hemp. A generic term covering all three varieties: Indica, Sativa and Ruderalis. It is derived from the Greek word "kannabis", from the areas of Thrace and Scythia. (The resulting overall botanical classification is Cannabaceae.) Cannabis refers to the entire plant, though only the buds, flowers and leaves are ingested for some desired effect. The balance of the plant is considered "vegetable matter" or "hemp", and can used for paper, rope, and other commercial products.

Cannabis Cup: The world's largest marijuana exposition, run by *High Times Magazine.* Started in 1988 by Steven Hager, it is held annually. It awards trophies in seventeen different marijuana-related categories.

cannaculture: The growing of marijuana.

cannaphobia: A state of mind common to those opposed to legalization.

cannon: A huge joint often containing up to four ounces of marijuana!

canoe: A badly burning joint, poorly rolled, with air pockets and seeds.

carb: Short for carburetor, it is the hole in a bong that clears the smoke out of the chamber between hits.

carrot bong: A bong created by strategically drilling three holes in a large carrot.

cashed: When a bong bowl is completely depleted with only ash remaining.

CBD oil: A concentrated oil produced from distilled cannabidiol-rich marijuana.

cannabinol (CBN): An important cannabinoid produced when THC breaks down in the body. It is not produced by the marijuana plant itself.

chalice: A Rastafarian Jamaican water pipe made from a coconut shell.

charas: Name given to marijuana resin in India, Nepal and Pakistan.

cheeba (or sheeba): Street slang for marijuana.

chimera: A plant with tissue from two genetically distinct parents.

chronic: Hip hop slang for ultra-potent marijuana. Also used in referring to "his chronic", meaning his repeated use of marijuana.

chuff: To cough without opening one's mouth.

cocaine: Chemically: benzoylmethyleogonine. A Schedule II street drug that is highly addictive and dangerous.

coffee shop: Netherlands. A one-stop shop for quality marijuana.

cola: Slang for the top flower cluster of a female marijuana plant.

collie: The top flower cluster of a female marijuana plant.

"Color" Reference: Telephone call code when you do not want to mention marijuana. "Did you get the green bike? Can I come over to check it out?"

concentrates: A product of the extraction of THC and CBD by any of a number of methods.

concrete: A botanical extraction including the plant's terpenes, waxes and lipids.

consemilla: A mature marijuana bud containing seeds.

cookie casualty: Slang expression for an overdose of any marijuana edible.

contact high: A high from breathing a nearby toker's exhaled smoke.

couchlock: Slang term for THC sedation without actual sleep.

crack: A cocaine derivative, often inhaled in the nose through a straw. In general in habitual users it produces toothless, wide-eyed, incoherent stuttering freaks. It is a Schedule I drug, *along with harmless marijuana!*

creeper: A marijuana high that sneaks up unexpectedly on a smoker.

crunchie: Derogatory slang for an environmentalist or liberal.

crutch: European slang, see British "roach".

crystal meth: The crystalline form of methamphetamine.

curing: The last stage in the marijuana drying process. Buds are placed in glass jars or wooden boxes for two to four weeks.

dab: A tiny rice-grain-size amount of concentrated marijuana extract.

dab rig: A type of water-filtration marijuana smoking pipe designed specifically for vaporizing concentrates.

dagga: African name for marijuana.

dank: The aroma of a strain is its "dank". Also slang for "really great" when referring to a particular strain.

deadhead: An habitual stoner. Often associated with an individual's affinity for music by the Grateful Dead.

dealer: The person supplying illegal marijuana or other street drugs.

dime bag: Ten dollars-worth of marijuana in a plastic baggie, almost always adulterated or of low quality

ditch weed: Low THC hemp plants that grow wild along

roadsides throughout the American Midwest. It is the "escaped" result of the government's WWII policy of encouraging mid-west farmers to grow hemp.

DL = "down low": A strategic discreet passing of a joint e.g. under-the-table. "Keep it DL dude."

draw: British slang, equivalent to American "stash".

dope: Generic term that refers to all illegal drugs.

dope rope: This is the slang term for common hemp-fiber cord and rope. It has been used by humans throughout history as sailboat rigging, and even earlier to tie together raft boards. Unfortunate drug connection attached to harmless hemp.

dry: "Out of". (I'm dry = I'm out of weed.)

dry sift: See kief.

dude: Term traceable to 1880s meaning a sharply dressed man. Presently a very common stoner term for a male or female, often implies a call to action: "Hey dude, check this out!" "Got any grass dude?" The female "dudette" never caught on.

Ecstasy: A common designer street drug that can (and often does) lead to hyperthermia, dehydration, kidney failure and heart failure.

edibles: Marijuana added to common food items such as brownies, doughnuts, cake, candy, pasta sauce ....just about anything. It does not act as rapidly as other forms of ingestion, and can lead to: "I guess I didn't eat enough of it". That decision can lead to ending up eating far more than needed with potentially unpleasant consequences. They also MUST be carefully kept out of the reach of children who are

315

drawn to sweets magnetically!

eighth: Slang for 1/8th ounce of marijuana.

Emerald Triangle: The area in northern California where conditions are optimal for the marijuana industry. Abundant sunshine, moderately warn temperatures, and a huge consumer base all contribute.

endocannabinoid: The natural cannabinoids produced in the human body (and all vertebrate animals) that regulate complex biological processes.

fatty: A particularly large joint.

fire: See "dank".

fluff: Light, airy buds, as opposed to dense buds.

flush the toilet: Good etiquette. After using a bong and before passing it, remove the stem and blow through it to clean it.

"Food" Reference: Telephone call code when you do not want to mention marijuana. "Come on over for dinner and bring the green veggies".

freshy: A nicely packed, all-green bong before the first hit.

fried: Feeling of complete intoxication.

funny cigarette: A marijuana joint.

fuzz: Street slang for police.

G-13: A pure cannabis Indica strain, almost tasteless but high in THC. Conspiracy theorists believe this was the first cannabis strain produced by the U. S. Government for research purposes.

gage: Jazz musician slang for marijuana ('30s & '40s).

ganja: Term for marijuana used in Asian India and Jamaica. It is believed the term has its origin in an ancient Sanskrit word.

genotype: The unique characteristics of a plant resulting from the combination of genes in the chromosomes present in any given plant.

grass: Common slang for marijuana.

greenhouse: Any outdoor building intended for marijuana growing that allows maximum sunlight to enter while allowing for control of the temperature, soil, water and atmosphere.

greenie: Derogatory slang for an environmentalist or liberal.

guano: Marijuana fertilizer. Bat poop, high in phosphorus. Sea bird poop, high in nitrogen.

hack: To steal, as in "hack your friend's stash".

"Harshed My Mellow": Someone adulterated my marijuana.

hash: Slang for hashish.

hash oil: An oil extracted from hashish by any of a number of processes.

hashish: A drug formed from the marijuana resinous heads' glandular trichomes. It is shaken or rubbed from floral clusters and pressed together and shaped by hand, often into balls. Can reach 55%+ THC content.

head shop: A retail establishment where one can purchase a wide variety of marijuana smoking accessories.

health stone: A porous ceramic filter used in the bowl of pipes used to smoke marijuana concentrates.

hemp: One of the four basic kinds of marijuana. Common name for ALL cannabis plants, but more specifically for those strains cultivated for non-medicinal industrial use. Derived from Old English "Haenep", it is the generic term for the roots, stalks and stems of any cannabis plant. Hemp is a potentially important commercial crop. It is essentially a "weed", fast growing, requiring no poisonous fertilizers and pesticides. It produces stronger paper than trees, obviating the need for huge pulp mills and their associated massive pollution.

herb: A common slang term for marijuana.

hempcrete: Concrete mixed with hemp fibers before pouring. Considered more durable, and it minimizes expansion-cracking.

hemp sheets: Slang for joint rolling papers made from 100% hemp fibers instead of commercial wood fibers. Paper made from pure hemp fibers is the most desirable. All other papers, the same as used in commercial tobacco cigarettes, may contain harmful chemicals when burned and inhaled.

heroin: A highly addictive substance that can, and often does, kill. Celebrities know to have died from a heroin overdose: John Belushi, Janis Joplin, Lenny Bruce, Chris Farley, Mitch Hedburg, and a host of others. Celebrities who have died from a marijuana overdose? **NONE.**

high: Feeling of complete intoxication.

holy roller: A joint rolled using paper torn from a bible, which is often similar to standard rolling papers.

homies: The folks you hang around with when you are smoking joints.

hookah (or hooka): A commonly-used mega-bong variant common in the Middle-East. One inhales through a hose which causes the lighted marijuana/tobacco mix to roast by drawing heat through burning charcoal at the top of the device. The smoke is filtered by the water through which it travels.

hookup: The person from whom you buy illegal marijuana.

honey oil: Hash oil.

horse (or "H"): Street slang for heroin.

hot box: What you have when you smoke marijuana in a car with the windows closed.

hubble bubble: A large Afghan water pipe used for smoking hashish.

huffing: Whether it is paint fumes, glue fumes, or magic marker fumes, straight from the sources or in paper bags, inhaling ("huffing") these substances is the quickest, easiest and cheapest "get high" drug any youth can buy. It can also kill.

Indica: One of the four basic kinds of marijuana.

Js: Slang for marijuana joints.

joint: A marijuana cigarette.

kali: Jamaican slang for top grade ganja.

KB: Kind bud.

key: Slang for a kilogram of a drug.

kief: See kif.

kif: A Moroccan word for hashish or marijuana. Also Moroccan term for a mixture of tobacco and marijuana.

kind: Kind bud.

kind bud: Slang for the best quality marijuana. Up to $800/ounce!

knife hit: Heat the tips of two butter knives, immediately press a small quantity of marijuana between the hot ends, inhale the smoke.

knock up: British slang for "to smoke" as in "let's knock up a spliff".

Kona buds: Marijuana from the Big Island of Hawaii.

krypto: Short for kryptonite.

kryptonite: Slang for the highest quality most potent strains of marijuana.

kush: A term broadly applied to high potency varieties of marijuana, most of which originated in the Hindu Kush region.

kutchie: Jamaican slang for a marijuana pipe. "Pass me da kuchie, mon."

laced: To be adulterated with a harmful substance.

Lamb's Bread: A classic Jamaican marijuana strain, named for colas the size of bread loaves!

land races: A generic term used to describe, as a group, the three pure THC producing varieties of marijuana: Indica, Sativa and Ruderalis. The original non-hybridized plants.

lit: Feeling of complete intoxication.

loaded: Feeling of complete intoxication.

magic mushrooms: Hallucinogenic wild mushrooms.

mari**h**uana: A spelling used in Mexico. First popularized by Harry Anslinger and William Randolph Hearst in their crusade to convince Americans of the dangers of this "Mexican scourge".

marajuana: A frequent *misspelling* of "marijuana".

marijuana: A term that refers specifically to the buds, flowers, and leaves of cannabis plants. It is Americanized Mexican Spanish.

maripills: Pill capsules, usually homemade, containing powdered marijuana.

MaryJane: Street slang for marijuana.

Maui Wowee: A classic '60s Sativa strain grown on Maui, Hawaii.

medibles: Short for "medicinal-edibles", brownies, etc.

medicinal cannabis: A generic term used to describe any marijuana-like cannabis-derived substance intended to treat some physical or mental illness. It is essentially the opposite of "recreational cannabis".

Mendocino Cigar: Usually a $1,000+ item made from the best quality marijuana rolled in a thin layer of bubble hash. Can require ten grams of hash and fourteen grams of buds!

mersh: Inexpensive street- marijuana. Any inferior marijuana product. Whatever crap a dealer can acquire and sell to individuals who are either nearly broke or don't know any better. This is often compressed Mexican marijuana glued together with Coca Cola, often containing mold and pesticides.

middles: Slang for a marijuana quality between Kind Bud (best) and mersh or schwag (worst).

mid-grade: See "middles".

mold: If marijuana is not properly "finished" and/or improperly packaged mold can form on the product. This is generally a white, thread-like mildew, which greatly affects the taste of the product, but is considered harmless. There is also a black-spot mold that can appear on buds.

mota: Mexican slang for marijuana.

muggles: 1920s slang for marijuana, common among jazz musicians.

munchies (the): The tendency for an individual under the influence of marijuana to have a craving for food, ANY food. Having a case of "The Munchies" often results in the over-consumption of junk food such as Twinkies, corn chips and potato chips, and can thereby lead to weight gain in heavy users.

"Music" Reference: Telephone call code when you do not want to mention marijuana. "Got any Marley CDs?"

mute: A homemade device for catching exhaled marijuana smoke.

nail: A small square of titanium or quartz which is heated with a torch. A drop of marijuana oil is then applied, instantly vaporizing it for inhalation

"Names" Reference: Telephone call code when you do not want to mention marijuana. "Did you see Jay (or Bud or Herb)

today".

narc: A slang term that applies to any law enforcement officer who might conceivably be enforcing federal or state marijuana laws.

Nederhash: Hash made from Dutch marijuana.

nickle bag: A five dollar bag of marijuana, the smallest unit sold. Offered in a plastic baggie, it is almost always adulterated or of low quality.

NLD: "Narrow Leaf Drug". Cannabis Sativa strain.

NORML: The National Organization for the Reform of Marijuana Laws, a major advocate for legalization of marijuana.

nudie: A single sheet of clear rolling paper.

nug: Short for nugget.

nugget: A high quality, properly cured, tight marijuana bud.

nug jug: A nug storage jar.

one hitter: A pipe meant for a single use before disposal.

oneie (won-ee): Slang for a one hitter.

opium: A narcotic created from poppies. It was extremely popular in the 1800s, and is still consumed in great quantities in the Near East.

oregano: A common Italian cooking herb. Because it has the exact appearance of crushed marijuana , and is a lot less expensive, it is often used to adulterate street-sold marijuana.

O.Z. (oh zee): Slang for one ounce of marijuana.

pakalolo: Hawaiian slang for marijuana; means "crazy tobacco".

Panama Red: Perhaps the most famous marijuana strain, originally from Central America. Its pure un-hybridized form produces a very strong psychedelic high. This *is* your grandpa's marijuana, far stronger than today's street product.

paraphernalia: A catchall term for devices for smoking marijuana, usually bought in a "head shop" or online.

PCP: Possibly the most dangerous addictive drug of them all. It creates in the user a sense of invincibility, and brings out truly animal-like aggressions.

peyote: A cactus derivative containing the hallucinogen mescaline. It is used by Mexican and American Indians in religious ceremonies.

phenotypes: Groups of observable marijuana characteristics such as smell, taste and effects on individuals.

phishhead: An habitual stoner.

psychedelic high: The effect produced by some marijuana strains and many other street drugs such as LSD where the user experiences weird dream-like experiences.

phytocannaboids: The plant version of endocannabinoids.

polm: Netherlands. Hashish produced by sifting dried marijuana flowers to capture the resin-filled trichrome heads, then pressing the heads.

polyphenols: The chemicals found in red wine. Studies have shown that THC and polyphenols affect the brain in a similar fashion, possibly keeping aging brains healthy and nimble.

pope: A homemade device designed to mask smoke odor. You exhale through a toilet paper roll tube that has a fabric softener sheet stuffed in one end.

pot: Generic slang term for marijuana.

pothead: Someone who smokes marijuana regularly.

potpreneur: An entrepreneur in the marijuana business.

pinch: To steal a small amount of marijuana that does not belong to you. It is pressed between the thumb and forefinger when reaching into a friend's bag of marijuana.

pinner: A very thinly rolled joint, easy to hide, fast burn, less smoke.

pull: Releasing the smoke from a bong chamber by lifting the stem from the base.

Q.P.: Slang for 1/4th pound or 4 ounces of marijuana.

quarter: Slang for 1/4th pound of marijuana, or 4 ounces.

Rasta Pasta: A spaghetti dinner served with a "special sauce". The sauce is made from any commercial jar sauce simmered for an hour or so with ground marijuana.

recreational cannabis (or recreational marijuana): A generic term for marijuana used for non-medical, personal pleasure.

reefer: A common slang term for a marijuana cigarette. It is derived from the Spanish word "grifa".

reefer madness: The term "reefer madness" was never heard in the United States before it was popularized and sensationalized in the 1936 release of the thoroughly moronic brainwashing propaganda movie "*Reefer Madness*".

resin (or rosin): The sticky exudation of the marijuana plant produced by its trichromes.

ripped: Feeling of complete intoxication.

rippers: Petty criminals who steal marijuana plants from private grow plots.

roach: American: The tiny bit left after a joint is fully smoked. British: A rolled up bit of business card or other thin cardboard used to hold a joint.

roach clip: A device for holding a joint so that when it burns down it doesn't burn your fingers.

Ruderalis: One of the four basic kinds of marijuana. A hardy variety of marijuana that is not dependent on environmental cues such as the light cycle to flower.

sack: Any bag of marijuana.

sack in: To pack ground marijuana into a bong's bowl.

Sativa: One of the four basic kinds of marijuana.

scissor hash: The resin that accumulates on tools used to remove leaf material in the preparation of dried marijuana.

scorch the bowl: A no-no. When smoking out of a pipe or bowl one should only light an edge and leave green for the next user.

schwag: Slang for the worst quality marijuana.

second generation joint: A joint rolled with debris from roaches.

shatter: One type of BHO, sold in thin, brittle, translucent sheets.

shotgun: A unique way to smoke a joint. One user carefully puts the lit end into their mouth, and blows smoke through the joint into the other's mouth, which contains the unlit end.

shrooms: Slang for magic mushrooms.

sinsemilla: Refers to seedless female marijuana flowers. Alternate meaning: Slang for any potent strain of marijuana.

skin: British slang for a rolling paper.

skin up: British slang for rolling a joint.

skunk: This is an Indica-Sativa cross with a highly sedating effect on the user. It is named after the animal whose defensive spray smells exactly like skunk-marijuana smoke! It was created in the 1970s by crossing Afghani and Indian marijuana strains. The original is "Skunk #1", but many hybrids have been created.

slide: The male part of a bong; goes into the female stem.

smoothie: Any mixed concoction of milk, cream, ice cream, fruit juices and marijuana. One writer claims great medicinal results from smoothies she makes using waste marijuana plant matter that she gets for free!

S.O.G. = Sea Of Green. Marijuana propagation with very tightly spaced plants giving small yield per plant but greatly conserving space.

sole: Flat sheets of hashish.

space cake: Any form of edible food containing marijuana.

spliff: British slang for a joint. American slang for a large joint.

stamen: The male floral organ which produces pollen.

stash: A marijuana users supply.

stem: The female part of a bong that accepts the slide.

stigma: The tip of a marijuana flower's pistil which receives the pollen.

stoned: Feeling of complete intoxication.

stone over: British slang for a marijuana hangover.

stoner: A heavy, long-time marijuana smoker.

strain: Any type of marijuana, as determined by its genetic makeup. A line of offspring plants derived from common ancestors.

sublingual: The method by which tinctures are placed under the tongue for absorption. It is faster acting than consuming edibles, but slower acting than smoking.

swayze: A clear rolling paper (named after Patrick Swayze in "Ghost".)

tall: "Getting tall" was a 1920s jazz musician term for getting "high" on marijuana.

tea: Jazz hipster slang for marijuana, used through the 50s. Current use: A cannabis recipe requiring boiling of ground marijuana in water. Because THC is not very water soluble boiling time should be longer than if using conventional tea leaves. Add some commercial tea later for flavor.

terpenes: The essential oils of all plants which creates their distinctive aromas.

Thai Sticks: Common way to import marijuana from Thailand. Buds and leaves are compressed and tied to a six-inch long bamboo stick, and sometimes dipped in opium.

THC: Technically "delta-9 tetrahydrocannabinol", the primary psychoactive agent in marijuana.

"Time" Reference: Telephone call code when you do not want to mention marijuana. "Can I come over for fifteen minutes (i.e., ¼ ounce wanted.") ....couple of hours (i.e., two ounces wanted.")

tincture: A marijuana preparation of powdered marijuana leaves or oil suspended in a solution, often glycerin or alcohol. It is administered sub-lingually (under the tongue) and is rapidly absorbed. It is a useful product for beginners because it is easy to take one drop at a time and watch for results. This can avoid an accidental overdose.

TNWLF: The National weed Legalization Fund, an advocate for legalization at: TNWLF.org or: https://www.thenationalweedlegalizationfund.org

toasted: Feeling of complete intoxication.

toke: To take a hit from a joint. (A toker is any weed smoker.)

top shelf: Slang for the best and most expensive strains of marijuana.

tracks: The marks (scars) left in the arms (and elsewhere) of heroin addicts from repeated injection needle use.

tree: An slang term for all marijuana plants. Possible origin is the fact that some marijuana plants can grow up to twenty feet high and could easily qualify as a "tree"!

trip: The effect of being high on a drug. The voyage on which the user of a strongly hallucinogenic drug such as LSD travels. (LSD trips can include engaging imaginary space monsters, dissolving walls, and jumping out of windows!)

trichromes: Specialized epidermal hairs. The cannabis plant gland heads where resin is produced. The THC-containing glands that grow off of marijuana buds and leaves.

vape: To vaporize and inhale marijuana or concentrates.

vape pen: A battery operated pen-sized micro-vaporizer, usually for BPOs, similar to an e-cigarette.

vegetable matter: The material left over, and often discarded, after the buds, flowers and leaves are removed. It can be "boiled down" (like maple sap in producing maple syrup) to produce a useful tea. It can also be used in "smoothies".

volcanoing: Slang term for accidentally *exhaling into* a bong and thereby exploding bong water and weed ash all over the place!

wacky tobaccy: Slang for marijuana.

wake and bake: To toke within an hour of rising in the morning.

wasted: Feeling of complete intoxication.

wax: A waxy substance resulting from a particular BPO method.

White Widow: A particularly powerful Indica/Sativa

crossbreed. Named for its whitish trichromes and its ability to incapacitate the user!

weed: Common generic term for marijuana.

Woodstock: A famous 1969 rock festival held in upstate New York.

wowee: Slang for Maui Wowee.

Yippies: Youth International Party members of a group started by stoners Abbie Hoffman, Jerry Rubin, and others.

Z (pronounced zee): Slang for one ounce of marijuana.

zonked: Feeling of complete intoxication.

zooted: Feeling of complete intoxication.

APPENDIX II
<u>MARIJUANA REFERENCE KNOWLEDGE</u>

This book is intended only as a general compilation of where we are at in the long drawn out process of educating the public (and especially educating our politicians) on the countless reasons why marijuana should be legalized both medicinally and recreationally.

A year ago one would have been hard pressed to find a single article on the internet or in print about *any* aspect of marijuana legalization efforts. Today you cannot search msn.com or yahoo.com or any other similar web-news area without finding at least one new article literally <u>every day</u>. *The legalization movement is in full gear throughout the country, and indeed throughout the world!*

The number of books available on the subject is impressive, numbering well over a hundred. The number of organizations dedicated to "spreading the word" has grown by leaps and bounds.

The author strongly urges anyone interested in learning everything there is to know about *"Marijuana – The Wonder Weed",* and in keeping up to the minute on legalization developments, avail themselves of the following resources:

<u>KEY MARIJUANA ORGANIZATIONS (there are many others a Google search will uncover):</u>

- Alliance For Cannabis Therapeutics (ACT) at: http://marijuana-as-medicine.org/alliance.htm

- Americans For Safe Access at: www.safeaccessnow.org

- Canadians For Safe Access at: http://safeaccess.ca

- Coalition For Cannabis Policy Reform at: ccpr.nationbuilder.com

- Common Sense for Drug Policy (CSDP) at: csdp.org

- Drug Policy Alliance (DPA) at: drugpolicy.org

- Drug Science Project at: www.drugscience.org

- Drug Sense at: drugsense.org

- European Coalition for Just and Effective Drug Policies (ENCOD) at: encod.org

- International Association For Cannabinoid Medicines at: www.cannabis-med.org

- Law Enforcement Against Prohibition (LEAP) at: www.leap.cc

- *Marijuana Business Daily* at: mjbizmedia.com

- Marijuana Legalization | The White House at: https://www.whitehouse.gov/ondcp/ondcp-fact-sheets/marijuana-legalizationo

- Marijuana Policy Project at: https://www.mpp.org/

- National Cannabis Industry Association at: thecannabisindustry.org \

- Teaching Seniors The Benefits of Cannabis at: thesilvertour.org

- The National Organization for Reform of Marijuana Laws (NORML) at: norml.org (and their many State Chapters and College Chapters).

- *The National Weed Legalization Fund at: TNWLF.org or https://www.thenationalweedlegalizationfund.org *An Arizona non-profit corporation started by the author in 2015.

- Vote Hemp at: www.votehemp.com

The author owes all of the above a debt of gratitude for providing much of the educational material offered to my readers in this book.

A SMALL SELECTION OF BOOK TITLES
<u>FROM MY PERSONAL LIBRARY</u>

The following are the books I found most useful in studying for and compiling the information for writing *MARIJUANA – THE WONDER WEED.* They represent only a fraction of my marijuana book library.

All are readily available on Amazon, both used and new. If you do not care to purchase them, any major library should have a copy of most of them.

I strongly suggest that you check out a selection of these books, especially if you are learning as much as possible in preparation for securing good employment in this rapidly expanding industry.

49 Business Ideas to Make Money in (Legal) Marijuana, By Megan Deal

Beyond Buds, by Ed Rosenthal

Book of Strains, by Justin Griswell & Victoria Young

Cannabinoids and Terpenes, by Ryder Management, Inc.

Cannabis Indica, Edited by S. T. Oner

Cannabis Pharmacy, by Michael Backes

Cannabis Sativa, Edited by S. T. Oner

CBD – Rich Hemp Oil, by Tina Rappaport & Dr. Steven Leonard-Johnson

Hallucinogens, by James Barter

Hemp for Health, by Chris Conrad

Marijuana Botany, by Robert Connell Clark

Marijuana Chemistry, by Michael Starks

Marijuana Growers Handbook, by Ed Rosenthal

Marijuana Horticulture, by Jorge Cervantes

Marijuana Medicine, by Christian Ratsch

Marijuana Smoker's Guidebook, by Matt Mernagh

The Benefits of *Marijuana*, by Joan Bello

Medical Marijuana 101, by Mickey Martin

Pot Culture, by Shirley Halperin & Steve Bloom

The Cannabis Grow Bible, by Greg Green

The Little Black Book of Marijuana, by Peter Pauper

The Medical Cannabis Guidebook, by Jeff Ditchfield & Mel Thomas

The Official High Times Pot Smokers Handbook, by David Bienenstock

The Pot Book, Edited by Dr. Julie Holland

Treating Holistically with Cannabis, by Marie J. Burke

Too High To Fail, by Doug Fine

Weed, by I. M. Stoned

I am not listing any of the large number of marijuana *cookbooks* I own. You can access dozens of cookbook titles through a Google or Amazon search for "Marijuana Cookbooks", "Cannabis Cookbooks", or "Pot Cookbooks". Many of the recipes are incredible!

APPENDIX III
MARIJUANA LAWS IN THE USA

Unfortunately, and disgracefully, United States federal law, against majority public opinion and all logic, still classifies marijuana in exactly the same "Schedule I Drug" as heroin and crack cocaine!

Our clueless government allows sale and use of the known killers alcohol and tobacco, along with hundreds of prescription drugs that are both addictive and deadly, but does not allow the sale and use of a harmless natural herb that has been shown for centuries to have curative effects on a wide variety of ailments. AND MARIJUANA DOES NOT KILL ITS USERS. It *cannot* kill.

Under **federal** law a first conviction for simple possession of any quantity of marijuana is punishable by up to one year in jail and a $1,000 fine. A second offense carries a minimum 15 day incarceration, with a maximum two years in prison and a maximum $2,500 fine. A third and any subsequent offenses carry a minimum jail time of ninety days up to a maximum of three year's incarceration and a $5,000 fine.

Do "Black Lives Matter"? Apparently not. Black youths are disproportionately affected by these Draconian laws. (See Chapter 34) Most important, these simple possession offenses follow an individual for the rest of their life and greatly limit future employment potential.

Worse are the federal penalties for selling marijuana or growing the plants. A first offense for even small quantities can put you in the slammer for five years. Large amounts carry a LIFE SENTENCE and a million dollar fine!

Remember, regardless of what the states are being allowed to do at present, our next President could, with a stroke of his or her pen, put every user, grower and seller in a concentration camp. There would be no space available in our already-overcrowded jails! Think this is impossible? Think again. It is reported by conspiracy theorists that many concentration camps are already sitting there staffed but empty!

Chris Christie, GOP one-time candidate for President and New Jersey Governor, has pledged publically that if elected he will put all dispensary owners in jail! It is not inconceivable that he could end up as Vice President, Attorney General, or the 9th Supreme Court justice. Then what?

The only candidate with a stated rational view on marijuana legalization is Bernie Sanders. He has mentioned full legalization!

In alphabetical order, here are the twenty-six (26) venues often quoted as being the ONLY places where marijuana is legal in varying degrees. They are noted below with the year of first legalization.

They are NOT, however, the ONLY venues where *some* medical exceptions also exist. To be entirely correct, FORTY-ONE different (out of a possible fifty-four major inhabited venues) allow SOME form of medical marijuana. (OK, I know there are sixteen United States Territories overall, but that includes eleven that are tiny and sparsely or entirely uninhabited so we can forget them!)

There is a massive variation among the different states as to the minute details of their marijuana laws. These many variables include at least the following:

- Medical use only, or medical and recreational use;
- Personal ID cards required or registration, and costs;

338

- What condition must the patient document to buy product?
- How much marijuana can a patient buy per month?
- How many plants can a patient self-grow?
- Licensing costs for each type of business (dispensary, grow, etc.);
- Who can get the various licenses?
- How many dispensaries are allowed?
- How many grow facilities are allowed?
- State and local taxes;
- How many doctors and which ones can document a patient's medical need?
- Housing restrictions;
- Employment restrictions;
- Custody disputes;
- Organ transplants;
- Legal age?
- What marijuana products are legal?
- Possession of x-ounces of buds at any time?
- Possession of x-ounces of leaves and plant matter;
- Possession of x-ounces of concentrate at any time;
- Possession of x-ounces of edibles at any time;
- Financial and jail-time penalties for excess possession;
- What delivery methods are legalized?
- DUI rules;
- Application fees;
- Licensing fees, initial and yearly;
- Excise taxes;
- Other taxes;
- Local cities' rules;
- Allowable number of grows and area;

- Allowable number of dispensaries;
- Allowable number of recreational retail stores;
- Allowable number of head shops;
- Decriminalization of small amount possession;
- Penalties for possession use, growing and sale.

When you realize all of the possible variables you can understand why a states such as Pennsylvania and Ohio, which legalized medical marijuana earlier in 2016, could well take over a year to finalize the details of their program. It is reported that it averages 18-24 months after a state "goes legal" for their program to be fully defined and implemented.

The twenty-six enlightened venues (twenty-five states plus the District of Columbia) each with its own comprehensive list of medical conditions that qualify an individual for a "medical marijuana card" are:

ALASKA: 1998. 1.0oz usable. 6 plants. One of the five venues allowing **FULL RECREATIONAL USE!** The Alaskan program did not get off to a great start! Apparently there is a lot of legal confusion about rules interpretation. For example, dues paying clubs are permitted where members are allowed to share and use marijuana, but they cannot sell marijuana.

ARIZONA: 2010. 2.5oz usable. 0-12 plants depending on proximity to a dispensary. Full recreational use may be approved by the public in November 2016.

The "Arizona Medical Marijuana Act" was approved 11/02/10 by 50.13% of voters. It was not until two years later on 11/15/12 that the first dispensary was licensed. A bill for full recreational use is expected to be on the ballot 11/16, and is expected to pass. (PTSD was finally added as a valid medical condition in early 2016.)

By July 7, 2016 Arizona marijuana advocates were require to get 150,642 valid signatures to get a measure on the November ballot making recreational marijuana legal (they planned to get over 230,000). This would allow possession of one ounce, and allow adults over 21 to cultivate up to six plants. There would be a15% tax at point of sale to the consumer.

Application fees are proposed to be $5,000. Fees could be as high as $30,000 for a grow facility, $15,000 to create various derivative products, $10,000 for testing facilities, $15,000 for medical dispensary distribution and $20,000 for recreational retailers.

At present there are about ninety legal dispensaries in the state. Marijuana social clubs will be permitted starting in 2020.

The two pro-recreational-use lobby groups are the *Marijuana Policy Project* and *Arizonans for Mindful Regulation.* Staunchly opposed to recreational use are the *Arizonans for Responsible Drug Policy.*

As an Arizonan I will be personally lobbying through my Arizona non-profit organization: The National Weed Legalization Fund (thenationalweedlegalizartionfund.org) and be monitoring our collective progress carefully.

CALIFORNIA: 1996 (The first state with medical legalization in America!) 8oz usable. 6 plants. Proposition 19 for recreational use failed in 2010. The new "Adult Use of Marijuana Act" will be up for a vote in 2016. 15% excise tax, 1oz +6 Plants, local cities can say NO to all. Existing dispensaries get first shot.

As with all things California nothing is ever straight forward or simple! There is potentially a bewildering number of ballot initiatives for November 2016. The Adult Use of Marijuana Act (AUMA) needs 365,880 signatures and is expected to achieve at least that number. That law would take effect January 1, 2018. (There is also a ballot initiative to allow full recreational use that will be voted on in November.)

That would give the state and individual cities lots of time to create oppressive rules and regulations! Local cities will be allowed to regulate or completely prohibit use.

There is a proposed 15% excise tax. Producers will pay a cultivation tax of $9.25/ounce of buds and $2.75/ounce of leaves. This may not seem like much, but it could preclude profitability!

In Los Angeles city by 2018 *all* medical dispensaries could be illegal. There is much complex legislation and counter-legislation being formulated. Major battles will be fought.

Without warning, and for no apparent reasons, MedWest in San Diego was raided by law enforcement authorities who seized computers, cash and products, and froze their bank account. It seems that throughout California there are many anti-marijuana forces at work!

COLORADO: 2000. 2oz usable. 6 plants. One of the five venues allowing **FULL RECREATIONAL USE! In** 2015 the state collected $135,000,000 in tax revenues on one billion dollars in marijuana product sales! Needless to say other states around the country are carefully watching Colorado. This is especially true regarding job creation. Over 17,000 occupational licenses were issued by the authorities in 2014. This figure was up to 27,000 in 2015.That's a lot of new jobs!

CONNECTICUT: 2012. "One month supply."   No home growing is permitted.

DISTRICT OF COLUMBIA: 2010. 2oz dry. One of five venues with **FULL RECREATIONAL USE** ! No home growing is permitted. The City Council voted 7- 6 earlier in 2016 to ban marijuana social clubs.

DELAWARE: 2011. 6oz usable. No home growing. With a $5,000 application fee and a $40,000 license fee (about the country-wide average) the state received eleven applications for the first two medical marijuana dispensaries.

HAWAII: 2000. 4oz usable. 7 plants.

Hawaii was the first state to legalize medical marijuana through the *legislative* process, back in 2000. In 2015 they passed the actual law authorizing sixteen medical marijuana dispensaries (six on Oahu (Honolulu), four on the Big Island (Kailua-Kona), four on Maui and two on Kauai.

How the sparse population on the latter two Islands could possibly support six dispensaries is beyond understanding. I predict that none of these dispensaries will ever show a profit, even if a federal reclassification to Schedule III allows normal corporate tax deductions. They may not open at all.

I lived in Hawaii for six years. There is probably more illegal marijuana grown in the Islands than anywhere else in America! It is literally everywhere and no one seems to care. This fact alone makes trying to run a profitable marijuana business a near impossibility. It is especially true because the local illegal product is top quality and inexpensive.

Aside from this, Hawaii's uber-high electricity costs will make profitable indoor cultivation virtually impossible. On top of that, inter-island transport of any marijuana product is illegal. Despite the potential challenges of running a marijuana business in Hawaii, 59 groups submitted 66 applications for the licenses. Back in late April 2016 Hawaii decided on which of 66 companies or individuals who had applied would be awarded licenses.

The Hawaii Department of Health required each winning applicant to pay a $75,000 licensing fee! They each also had to show they have $1,000,000 *cash* reserves *plus* $100,000 for each dispensary location. Dispensaries were permitted to begin operations by July 15th. A lack of testing labs, required on each Island, could create a problem and delay implementation indefinitely. Each winner will be allowed to open up to two cultivations and two dispensaries.

The applicants were a very eclectic mix of individuals and groups. The list include a retired two-star U.S. Navy Admiral, a local surfing legend, **Henk Rogers** (the developer of a blockbuster video game) and Woody Harrelson, actor and a marijuana legalization activist. One group even has former Surgeon General Kenneth Moritsugu on its team! The applicant list also included lawyers, physicians, educators and a businessman specializing in tourism and hospitality.

It is interesting to note that **Union Local 480 (food related)** struck a deal with Green Aloha, a Kauai-based company seeking a medical marijuana license. Unions nationwide are getting excited over the huge numbers of citizens who will eventually be employed in this fledgling industry.

Unfortunately Woody Harrelson did not win a license. Neither did Henk Rogers.

ILLINOIS: 2013. 2.5oz usable every 14 days. No home growing.

The marijuana industry in Illinois is struggling. Although medical marijuana has been legal since 11/09/15, and there are at present 22 licensed dispensaries with more to open in 2016, only a *scant 4,000 patients* have been granted access. About as many have pending applications. The industry claims it needs as many as 30,000 patients to be viable. So why is the number of patients so low?

For one, many doctors are still totally under the influence of Big Pharma and simply will never prescribe marijuana. If it isn't the perks they get, it is also a fear that, because marijuana is still federally illegal, and a Schedule I drug, there may be some unexpected federal legal liability.

Most important is the very limited list of medical conditions that marijuana is approved for in Illinois. The biggest "missing ailment" is "chronic pain" which can be due to everything from common arthritis to accident trauma, to irritable bowel syndrome, and a host of other common ailments.

The state of Illinois was, however, the first enlightened authority when it comes to PTSD vets and marijuana (followed recently by Arizona.). A bill was passed that allows veterans to circumvent doctor participation in obtaining marijuana permits. Instead, veterans can directly petition the Illinois State Department of Health for review of their medical records.

The *Marijuana Legalization Act* will be on the ballot in November 2016. It calls for no employment discrimination for legal users. There will be low license fees. But cultivation will be limited to just 800,000sqft for the entire state, which is quite low...that's only 20 acres! There was that much being grown in my small Hawaii neighborhood!

If a hard-core group of marijuana-hating politicians get out of the way, and the Illinois Health Department wakes up and approves marijuana for all of the conditions it has been proven to help, Illinois could be a major legalization success story in the future.

MAINE: 1999. 2.5oz. 6 plants.

There is a ballot initiative to allow full recreational use that will be voted on in November 2016

License fees for retail stores will be only $2500. Laboratories will be charged just $500, and social clubs, which *are* allowed, will pay only $2,500.

MARYLAND. 2014. "30 day supply" (This was recently defined as ten ounces every two weeks). No home growing.

MASSACHUSETTS: 2012. "60 day supply". 6 plants permitted. There is a ballot initiative to allow full recreational use that will be voted on in November 2016.

The *REGULATION AND TAXATION OF MARIJUANA ACT* sadly offered no housing or employment protections.

Because of low crop yields the state is experiencing shortages. A recreational marijuana initiative seems to be suffering from a lack of interest and political activity on the part of present dispensary owners.

MICHIGAN: 2008. 2.5oz usable. 12 plants. A ballot initiative to allow full recreational use that was to be voted on in November 2016 was shot down by the governor for insufficient signatures within a newly specified time limit.

MINNESOTA: 2014. 30dy supply NON-smokeable. No home growing.

MONTANA: 2004. 1oz usable. 4 plants.

This has become the "model *problem* state". There are dozens of legally operating dispensaries. But the Montana Supreme Court said that the entire medical marijuana program must be eliminated by August 2016! Every dispensary can service THREE PATIENTS TOTAL, or be shut down. The Montana Cannabis Industry Association has asked for delays and has been granted a few.

BUT, the United States Supreme Court in June refused to hear an appeal which means the Montana Supreme Court ruling stands! If dispensaries are only allowed to service three individual patients each, profitability is impossible.

Is this the absolute end of the medical marijuana movement in Montana? No, the public could still vote on a program in the future. In fact, there is a ballot initiative to allow full recreational use that will be voted on in November 2016!

But will this give pause to ANY potential dispensary owners in Montana, and perhaps nationwide in the future? Very possibly so. It is a *very* bad precedent.

NEVADA: 2000. 1oz usable. 7 plants (but legislation eliminated *all* growing facilities as of 03/01/16.) *The Initiative to Regulate and Tax Marijuana* will finally take effect in January 2017.

There is a ballot initiative to allow full recreational use that will be voted on in November 2016.

Nevada charges $5,000 for a dispensary application and $20,000 for the license. Laboratory licenses are $15,000, grow operations $30,000. Product creation facilities will pay $10,000. There will be a 15% excise tax on all sales.

There is no protection against discrimination in housing or at the workplace. Worse, the DUI provision is onerous. Most states require some degree of obvious impairment. Nevada only requires the *presence* of marijuana in a car for an arrest!

High Times Magazine seeks to build a new casino in Las Vegas that will permit smoking marijuana on the premises. They already have their cabaret and gaming licenses in place.

NEW HAMPSHIRE: 2013. 2oz usable every 10 days. No home growing.

NEW JERSEY: 2010. 2oz usable. No home growing. The program is faltering because of low crop yields and product shortages. Having an anti-legalization Governor cannot help.

NEW MEXICO: 2007. 6oz usable. 16 plants. Special license is needed to home-grow.

NEW YORK: 2014. 30 day supply, must be NON-smokeable. No home growing.

New York has had a very slow ramp-up of their medical marijuana program. Only roughly two-thousand patients have been certified as needing medical marijuana. Of these, only half have ever set foot in one of the scant five dispensaries which are very widely separated geographically.

OHIO: Legislation failed in 2015, despite a major effort, but has since been passed. Dispensaries were to become licensed in early 2016. In preparation for licensing, some dispensaries ramped up in anticipation of a fast start. Bad idea! The police raided a number of these new potential dispensaries who were in the process of setting up their operations prior to licensing, which they thought was only a few weeks away. They literally demolished the operations! A nice way for the medical marijuana program to begin!

BUT soon after, in June, Governor Kasich signed Bill 523 making medical marijuana fully legal for a full range of illnesses!

OREGON: 1998. 24oz usable.   24 plants. (That's a *lot* of plants!) One of five venues allowing **FULL RECREATIONAL USE!**

The first measures to legalize marijuana began way back in 1982! In 2013 the Oregon Legislature regulated medical dispensaries. Officially full legalization took place on July 1, 2015.

Oregon suffers from hyper-regulation, with separate licensing for medical and recreational dispensaries, along with separate sets of rules. Owners and *investors* MUST be Oregon residents. Myriad laws regulating everything imaginable are making it difficult for growers and dispensaries to stay in business.

New restrictions on the number of patients who can register at a given grow site are confusing matters further. There are NO license caps in Oregon. At this writing there are around 600 applications pending for grow operations, 150 for retail stores, 70 for infused product makers, and 4 for testing labs. There are around 330 licensed medical marijuana dispensaries presently in operation.

Oregon is the only venue that allows customers from other states to buy marijuana. They also allow their medical dispensaries to sell edibles and concentrates to recreational users.

PENNSYLVANIA: 2016 (effective 2017 - 2018). Details not yet decided. Apparently no smoking or marijuana growing will be permitted.

RHODE ISLAND: 2006. 2.5oz usable. 12 plants. The state may soon be joining the growing list of states that add PTSD as a covered illness.

VERMONT: 2004. 2oz usable. 9 plants. The governor has come out in favor of recreational marijuana. Bernie Sanders home state is well known as the most liberal in America.

WASHINGTON: 1998. 24oz usable. 15 plants. One of five venues allowing **FULL RECREATIONAL USE!**

The state's 2105 sales revenue was $257,000,000, with taxes collected equaling seventy million dollars.

The biggest operational problem faced by the marijuana growing industry in Washington (and for that matter nationwide) is the complex federally mandated seed to sale tracking. A company called BioTrack THC created an inventory tracking software product that the state adopted at the time of legalization. They won the very lucrative contract over a number of other software companies.

It is reported that Washington growers describe the software system as a "time suck and a nightmare". It is almost universally hated. There is a free version, and a "bells and whistles" version that costs about $400/month. Neither one is popular.

Apparently it takes too much time to use, and time is money. It is just one of the many obstacles set up by a government that seems to do everything possible to slow down full implementation.

It is over-regulation, and the added costs passed on to the marijuana consumer that has the cartels licking their chops. Unfettered by regulations they can offer marijuana at prices far under those that a legal dispensary can offer.

The Washington State Liquor and Cannabis Board has cracked down on growers using poisonous pesticides. They are shutting down grow facilities where they simply *see* pesticide canisters that they consider illegal. As of July 1, 2016 *all* medical marijuana will be tested for pesticide residue. The Washington Department of Agriculture has created a list of pesticides approved for use.

The following are the sixteen additional states (for forty-one total states, forty-two venues including D.C.) that can honestly say: "We presently have a medical marijuana law on the books." These laws apply to **CBD oil only**, and are very restrictive as to the conditions that can be treated. But it's a small start on the long road to universal decriminalization and legalization.

In five of these states the laws are named specifically for one individual child who has clearly benefited from the use of CBD oil to control spasticity.

ALABAMA: 2014. "Carly's Law".

The state has some of the nation's harshest marijuana penalties, and the most unjustly applied laws. Although blacks and whites are shown to use marijuana at about the same per capita rate, blacks are 4.4 times more likely to be arrested for marijuana "crimes". In 2015 there were very modest reductions in possession penalties

Although 75% of Alabamans support medical legalization, a medical marijuana bill could not even find a hint of legislative support.

FLORIDA: 2014. CBD for epileptic seizures and cancer. There is a ballot initiative up for a November 2016 vote that could expand the diseases covered.

In 2014 billionaire casino mogul Sheldon Adelson derailed legalization legislation. The bill fell just short of 60% needed to pass. At present it is reported that 65% are in favor of decriminalization. It is expected to pass in the 2016 November elections. Orlando decriminalized carrying small amounts of marijuana. Tampa did likewise back in April 2016.

GEORGIA: 2015. "Haleigh's Hope Law".

IOWA: 2014. CBD for epilepsy.

KENTUCKY: 2014. CBD for epilepsy.

MISSISSIPPI: 2014. "Harper Grace's Law".

MISSOURI: 2014. CBD for epilepsy. There is a ballot initiative for a wider range of diseases to be voted on in November 2016.**NORTH CAROLINA**: 2014. CBD for epilepsy.

OKLAHOMA: 2015. CBD for epilepsy. There is a ballot initiative for a November 2016 vote to greatly expand the illnesses covered.

SOUTH CAROLINA. 2014: "Juliens Law".

TENNESSEE: 2014. CBD for seizures.

TEXAS: 2015. CBD for epilepsy.

Texas COULD become a FULL LEGALIZATION STATE based on the November 2016 election results! The deeply conservative tea-party backed David Simpson, House Republican, explained in an op-ed that his belief in GOD, distrust in government, and criticism of the "War On Drugs" led him to sponsor a marijuana legalization bill. He is quoted as saying:

"As a Christian I recognize the innate goodness of everything GOD made and humanity's charge to be stewards of the same. I don't believe that when GOD made marijuana he made a mistake that government needs to fix."

Medical marijuana in Texas has been limited to CBD for epilepsy. It is estimated that 150,000 Texans are epilepsy sufferers. It is planned that there will be twelve dispensary licenses issued in 2017. There is a movement to expand the covered ailments before that time.

UTAH: 2014. "Charlee's Bill". CBD for epilepsy.

VIRGINIA: Passed a *very* narrow law in 2015 relating to epilepsy.

Although 86% of Virginians want medical marijuana, there is no strong legislative initiative. Law enforcement is strongly against any legalization because of DUI concerns. (Or maybe they are afraid they won't have as many black kids to arrest?)

WISCONSIN: 2014. CBD approved under strict conditions.

LAST, we have the ten troglodyte knuckle-dragging states and the five inhabited territories which apparently have their heads so buried in the sand that legalizing marijuana simply scares the hell out of them for no sound reason. (Actually, many of these have at least made some effort to introduce legislation in the past.) These are:

ARKANSAS: "The Arkansas Medical Cannabis Act" was certified by the Attorney General in September 2014. It will be on the ballot in November 2016, if at least 67,887 valid signatures are obtained.

IDAHO: "Alexis' Law" failed in 2015. Poor Alexis. The GOP controlled legislature by a vote of 29-5 passed a measure declaring marijuana to be: "unhealthy, unsafe, addictive and debilitating EVEN WHEN USED FOR MEDICINAL PURPOSES." Sadly out of touch morons.

INDIANA: I am an ice cube. I just found myself in Hell. I am a potential marijuana entrepreneur living in Indiana. Same chance. Legislation failed in 2015. Senator Karen Tallian's "Compassionate Medical Marijuana" bill did not even advance as far as receiving a hearing!

KANSAS: Legislation failed in 2015. Seventy percent of Kansans support medical marijuana. Two Senators, David Haley and Gail Finney offered medical marijuana bills. They received almost no legislative support.

LOUISIANA: In 2015 penalties for possession and use were revised slightly downward. But legalization of any kind is a far future dream. Yet another doomed ice cube!

NEBRASKA: Legislation failed in 2015. Although there is definite legislative sentiment, Governor Ricketts indicated that he opposes medical marijuana. (Can medical marijuana cure rickets?) Lawmakers warned that approving marijuana without the U. S. Food and Drug Administration's blessing could have "consequences". "It is a dangerous position for legislators to practice medicine." Chickens!

NORTH DAKOTA: Legislation failed in 2015. A bi-partisan group of seven Senators introduced a medical marijuana bill. It died in the House. Next session? 2017. There is a possibility that it could make the ballot in November 2016 if the required number of signatures are received.

SOUTH DAKOTA: There is no active interest shown in any legislative incentives towards marijuana for any purpose whatsoever. Hell's getting wetter!

WEST VIRGINIA: Legislation failed in 2015. Although public support is up to 56%, various medical marijuana bills failed to advance through the legislature. It is expected that the next session could see passage of something positive.

WYOMING: There appears to be no legislative interest in passing any sort of marijuana legalization any time soon. And wetter still!

AMERICAN SAMOA: This territory has problems with amphetamines and wide spread marijuana use. It has some of the strictest penalties for possession and use (a classic example proving that penalties themselves are almost pointless.) There is no initiative for legalization of any kind.

GUAM: A successful ballot initiative actually legalized medical marijuana in this territory. A 151 page document has outlined all of the provisions, and there will be public hearings "sometime" in the future before the plan is implemented.

NORTHERN MARIANA ISLANDS: Marijuana is illegal for any purpose. There have, however, starting in 2015, been a number of proposals that are being discussed that could change this position in the future.

PUERTO RICO: In 2013 a medical marijuana bill failed in the legislature. In 2015 Governor Padillo to the surprise of many signed an executive order to authorize the use of medical marijuana in the territory. There is considerable support, but details of any plan are far from completed. It is possible that at some time in late 2016 medical marijuana will finally be legal in the territory. They BADLY need the tax revenue!

Considering the massive financial woes on the Island, I cannot imagine the potential tax revenue not being a huge incentive for full legalization and "marijuana tourism".

VIRGIN ISLANDS: Marijuana is widely available in the territory. Possession of small quantities has been decriminalized, but legislation has yet to be formulated. Governor DeJongh is a strong opponent of legalization, and it took a veto override to get decriminalization on the books.

So, if anyone ever asks you the trivia question: "How many states have laws on the books legalizing medical marijuana?" what would you now answer? The correct answer is "**Forty-ONE**"! "How may *venues*?" "Forty-two"! Very few individuals with whom I have spoken can answer this question correctly.

It is a fact that almost ninety percent (90%) of the United States population presently resides in a state that has at least *some* medical marijuana legislation on the books! I have never seen this figure published anywhere else.

About half of all Americans presently live in states with comprehensive medical marijuana laws in place.

Incredible as it may seem to some, there are active movements in two states where medical marijuana is presently legal to have it available to <u>elementary school nurses</u> to administer to grade-school kids as needed! This has *already happened* in New Jersey, and by the time you read this it will likely be true in Colorado. Baby steps towards ultimate legalization success? Let us hope so.

Even in states where recreational use is legal, there can be serious penalties for possession of large amounts at any given time. For example, in Colorado if you are found to have more than 12 ounces of marijuana you could face two years in jail and a $100,000 fine! You can also be fined $1,000 just for smoking a joint in public.

Oregon is not quite as expensive as Colorado. Possession of a pound and a half of marijuana would only set you back just $5,000 and put you in the slammer for a year! Public smoking will set you back $600.

In Washington state possession of 2 ½ ounces or more is going to set you back $10,000, and potentially incarcerate you for five years! They don't fool around in Washington! But smoking in public is only a $100 fine, so it's not all bad.

It is almost impossible to keep up fully with all of the new initiatives and law changes, which are quite frequent. I suggest you get a free internet e-mail subscription to the *Marijuana Business Daily* (mjbizmedia.com). Here you will be kept appraised of most state changes as they occur.

SUGGESTION: If you have any hope of EVER being able to use marijuana legally for any purpose, move from, or never move to, Indiana, Louisiana, South Dakota, Wyoming or American Samoa! (Compliments of Anderson Travel Advisory Services!)

APPENDIX IV
<u>MARIJUANA LAWS WORLDWIDE</u>

International marijuana laws are not "cut and dried", but somewhat vague. They are covered under Section IV of the "Single Convention on Narcotic Drugs" (thank you again, Harry Anslinger) which subjects marijuana to various suggested restrictions. It was signed in 1961 by 181 countries. Article 2 of the Convention states:

"A Party shall, if in its opinion the prevailing conditions in its country render it the most appropriate means of protecting the public health and welfare, prohibit the production, manufacture, export and import if, trade in, possession or use of any such drug except for amounts which may be necessary for medical and scientific research only, including clinical trials therewith to be conducted under or subject to the direct supervision and control of the Party."

That's quite a long sentence! One could interpret it as totally excluding recreational use of marijuana. One could also conclude that any country which considers recreational use an *"appropriate means of protecting the public health and welfare"* can deregulate marijuana as it sees fit. Some have. Many have not.

The *United Nations General* Assembly *Special Session On Drugs* known by the acronym "UNGASS" (you can't make this stuff up!) met in April 2016. Originally scheduled for 2019, it was decided by members to hold this Special Session annually instead of once every ten years. And "ungas" they did, in a typical bureaucratic circle-jerk! The progress they made is summed up on UNGASS' official website: "Defenders of the status quo have prevented any effective changes in

358

the global drug problem". Ninety-three nations voted. As "us" Brooklyn Dodgers ('Dem Bums) rabid baseball fans used to say: **"Wait 'till next year!"**

There are approximately 220 countries worldwide. Only four allow legal sale of marijuana for *both* medical *and* recreational use. These are Bangladesh, Germany (with licensing), North Korea (which, as far as known, has no marijuana regulation statutes) and Uruguay. Two countries, Cambodia and Cyprus have decriminalized the sale of marijuana.

In the Netherlands only special "coffee shops" can sell marijuana. Amsterdam has been for years the world's "Marijuana Capital".

Though technically illegal, marijuana sales are *tolerated* in India, and are legal in certain cities in Canada. In Canada a recreational marijuana bill is expected in 2017. Prime Minister Trudeau is leaning towards a very liberal position.

In the "nothing in the marijuana industry is ever certain (think Montana) category", Vancouver's new stricter regulations could close as many as 150 dispensaries, leaving as few as 35 operating under a set of newly revised statutes.

In India's Muslim culture smoking hashish in a hookah is a regular part of daily life. Hindus, especially the Brahman caste, often smoke marijuana products for relaxation. Marijuana based drinks are sold in government authorized "bhang shops" in the northern India cities of Varansi, Puri, Jaiselmer, & Pushbar.

Goa on India's west coast is a known mecca for marijuana smokers. Indian hash (charas) from Nepal, rolled spliff style with tobacco, is smoked openly everywhere.

Speaking of Nepal, marijuana was legal there through the '70s. Now technically illegal, it is widely tolerated everywhere.

Seven other countries allow sale for medical purposes *only*, with varying restrictions: Chile, Columbia, Croatia, Czech Republic, Finland, Israel and Serbia.

Croatia legalized medical marijuana in 2015.

In The Czech Republic, and in Prague in particular, authorities are extremely lenient in enforcing any marijuana laws.

The laws on transporting marijuana essentially follow the laws for sales in almost every country.

There is only **one** country on the planet where there are, by stated law, no limits on the possession, use, sale, transport and cultivation of marijuana. It is 100% legal for ANY purpose. That country is **Uruguay**. Hooray for Uruguay! (Full availability was scheduled for June 2016.)

It should be noted that, to the disappointment of the anti-marijuana crowd, there has been absolutely **NO ADDITIONAL CRIME IN URUGUAY SINCE LEGALIZATION!** But the program is new, and will be watched carefully.

Two other countries have no laws on the books that prohibit marijuana use, sale, transport or cultivation of marijuana. These countries are **Bangladesh** and **North Korea**.

Every other country on the planet has some level of restrictions. A few countries are at the absolute *opposite* end of the scale from Uruguay.

For example, in 2002 The Philippines' President Macapagal-Arroyo signed into law a *mandatory* **DEATH PENALTY** for all drug dealing in _any_ amount. If you are planning on dealing dime bags of marijuana don't go there!

In Malaysia, if you are caught and convicted of trafficking illegal drugs you will be subject to a **MANDATORY death sentence**! As of 2015 there are over a thousand prisoners on death row awaiting hanging! In a famous case a single mother was sentenced to death for possessing just 18 grams (0.64oz) of marijuana. These guys just don't fool around!

HINT: Avoid Malaysia and The Philippines! Just imagine: Some wise-ass casually dropping a joint into your pocketbook or your pants pocket could be fatal! Of course, anyone familiar with the movie _Midnight Express_ might also hesitate before taking a vacation in beautiful historic Turkey!

There are many countries where the marijuana laws are pretty loose. Germany, Belgium, The Netherlands, the Czech Republic, Italy and Portugal in Europe, and Peru, Columbia and Brazil in South America fall into this category.

Portugal has had great success over the past fifteen years with a comprehensive harm-reduction strategy. Non-violent drug offenders are kept out of jail and subjected to mandatory marijuana education. Use is down by 50% overall!

Twenty-six countries have officially decriminalized possession for varying small quantities up to _all_ amounts **(ARE YOU LISTENING USA?)**:

Argentina, Australia (certain states), Austria, Belgium, Bolivia, Cambodia, Chile, Columbia, Costa Rica, Croatia, Cypress, Czech Republic, Ecuador, Estonia, Greece, Italy Jamaica, Jordan, Malta, Mexico, Peru, Portugal, Russia, Slovenia, Spain, Switzerland and Ukraine.

Countries where marijuana is still illegal, but *fully* decriminalized include:

Austria, Bolivia, Cambodia, Chile, Costa Rica, Croatia, Cyprus, Estonia, Italy, Jamaica, Jordan, Mexico, Slovenia, Spain and Switzerland.

Until recently in Costa Rica it was permitted to grow some marijuana plants, but the government has begun to crack down on large grows in particular.

In Jamaica, marijuana is grown everywhere. This is primarily because of the almost-universal Rastafarian religion, which considers the herb to be sacred. Marijuana is technically illegal, but if you happen to be there and an arrest seems imminent, "Don't worry; Be Happy". The police are easily bribed!

Countries where small amount are decriminalized, but marijuana is still illegal, are: Argentina, Belgium, Columbia, Czech Republic, Ecuador, Greece, Malta, Peru, Russia, and The Ukraine.

Belize, India and Columbia simply tolerate marijuana use, even though it is technically illegal. The same is true in India for the sale, transportation and growing of marijuana.

In Germany, possession is legal "with permission", and the sale, transport and cultivation are fully legal!

In France, especially in Paris, smoking marijuana is illegal, but common and widely tolerated.

In Denmark, there is an area known as "The Amsterdam of Scandinavia". It is located within Copenhagen. It is a self-governing neighborhood called Christiana.

There are six countries where *growing* marijuana plants can be a legal enterprise, some with restrictions: Bangladesh, Germany, Jamaica, North Korea, Spain and Uruguay. In Canada small quantities being grown are tolerated almost everywhere.

Although still illegal, growing marijuana has been *decriminalized* in sixteen countries: Australia (some states), Belgium, Cambodia, Chile, Columbia, Costa Rica, Cypress (hemp only), Czech Republic, Jordan, Malta, Mexico, The Netherlands, Portugal, Russia, Slovenia and Ukraine.

It is quite apparent that growing marijuana plants takes place in MANY countries where growing is technically illegal. Just look at some of the published studies of various worldwide strains that have been conducted. Plants grown from seed from 50+ countries have been studied!

Countries producing marijuana seed (illegally) include: Switzerland, Brazil, Cyprus, Columbia, Costa Rica, Ghana, Iran, Lebanon, Pakistan, Afghanistan, Nepal, Morocco, Chile, Czechoslovakia, Ethiopia, Israel, Manchuria, France, Poland, Greece, Italy, Peru, Bulgaria, Russia, and Yugoslavia.

Add to these Thailand, Turkey, England, Ireland, Argentina, Gambia, India, Japan, Korea, Mexico, Netherlands, South Africa, Sweden , Vietnam, Hungary, Romania, Paraguay, Senegal, and Sierra Leone.

So, regardless of the United Nations edict, marijuana is literally grown worldwide!

In April 2016 Mexico's President Enrique Pena Nieto announced that his country would move soon to legalize medical marijuana. There is no specific date for implementation.

Considered illegal in England, marijuana is widely available and used on University campuses. This is not unlike extensive use in American colleges. Remember the famous Turf Tavern at Oxford University? This is where Rhodes Scholar William Jefferson Clinton famously "did not inhale"! At least President Obama admitted: "Of course I inhaled. That was the idea."

In England there is only one single place where marijuana can be legally grown. This is the property owned by GW Pharmaceuticals, featured in a recent television documentary. Operating under a special license they have developed "Sativex" for treating multiple sclerosis. Sativex spray is available by prescription in Canada, New Zealand, the United Kingdom, Germany, Spain & Denmark.

Countries presently studying Sativex are: Italy, Sweden, Austria, The Czech Republic, Belgium, Finland, Iceland, Ireland, Luxemburg, The Netherlands, Norway, Portugal, Poland & Slovakia. The United States has actually begun to test Sativex as well. One reported issue with Sativex is that a two week supply costs in excess of two-hundred dollars!

Australia is pushing to be at the forefront of medical marijuana studies. In 2015 the Australian government announced that it would be allowing cultivation of medical marijuana. Federal Health Minister Susan Ley has put her support behind legislation that would allow her agency to oversee the growing and eventual clinical trials.

"Currently there are already systems in place to license the manufacture and supply of medicinal marijuana - based products in Australia. There is no mechanism in place to allow the production of a safe, legal and sustainable local supply." Ms. Ley said. Three Australian states – New South Wales, Victoria and Queensland – quickly joined in and pledged to hold clinical trials for patients suffering from terminal illnesses, those undergoing chemotherapy and children with severe epilepsy.

Many Australian states will likely view this as a way to recover from shrinking tax revenues. Australia could well be the start of a new major medical marijuana market. Australian medical cannabis company MMJ PhytoTech Ltd. has just sold its first marijuana pills via a Swiss-based subsidiary. The bad news: The pills are only available in Europe. (Ten milligrams cost around $130, not exactly inexpensive.)

While medical marijuana remains by and large illegal in Australia, a survey from Palliative Care Australia recently learned that 67% of Aussies would be fine with patients using some form of marijuana to help with chronic pain and illness. AusCann, an Australian marijuana producer, was awarded a license earlier this year to grow medicinal marijuana on Norfolk Island and export it to Canada.

I know personally of a young female PhD candidate researcher in Sydney who is studying the marijuana constituent "terpenes", an area that has not been well researched.

In the northeast corner of New South Wales, 500 miles north of Sydney, there is a major marijuana-smoker hippie-heaven! The annual "Mardi Gras & Drug Reform Rally" is held there, with stoners from all over the region in blissful attendance.

Israel is clearly light years ahead of the United States in studying medical marijuana, and in recognizing its value as a potent medicine. Two major Israeli ***hospitals*** have actually installed marijuana vaping equipment for their patients in need of pain and nausea relief! Want to take a guess when the first hospital in the United States will do that? My guess is "maybe" by 2030. Maybe never.

Scientists at the Technion Israel Institute of Technology in Haifa recently released the first results of a cancer study that examined the effects of <u>50 varieties of marijuana</u> with 200 different cancer cells. They found the results promising, and are continuing their research to this day. (NOTE that I said **"50 varieties".**)

All United States studies are presently limited to the **ONE STRAIN OF MARIJUANA,** grown legally at the University of Mississippi. This is a perfect example of why, unless our government wakes up and stops dragging out marijuana studies forever, we will never catch up to other countries worldwide.

Marijuana is technically illegal in Israel but the local police have a lot more important things to worry about, like Palestinians, missiles, and a future nuclear-bomb armed Iran, to name just a few!

Back in '09 there was an unsuccessful push for Knesset seats by a group calling itself the "Holocaust Survivors' and Grown-Up Green Leaf Party". They failed to win a single seat! Better luck next time.

Travelers to anywhere outside of the United States must familiarize themselves with the drug laws in every country they plan to visit. This includes legal prescription drugs as well. Get something in writing from the local Consulate office prior to departure.

The best policy is to **NEVER CARRY DRUGS OF ANY KIND INTO A FOREIGN COUNTRY.** Laws change. Corruption is rampant among law enforcement in many places.

<u>Don't tempt fate!</u>

APPENDIX V
AN OPEN LETTER
TO PRESIDENT OBAMA

THE *BEST* SOLUTION TO
PRESIDENT OBAMA'S LEGACY PROBLEMS

Dear President Obama:

The 2016 election is approaching rapidly. Heaven help any 2016 presidential candidate who comes out in favor of stricter marijuana enforcement! Even openly standing for the status quo would be catastrophic, as would be simply ignoring the public outcry for federal decriminalization and legalization.

Some candidate other than Senator Bernie Sanders needs to have the courage to call for full legalization of marijuana if they hope to win in November.

Be it a Republican (are you listening Donald?) or Democrat (are you listening Hillary?) if either runs on a platform of decriminalizing marijuana, and full federal legalization, young voters nationwide, and many older voters too, who would never otherwise even *show up* at the polls will flock to that candidate in droves and *insure a solid victory*!

But why wait for November 2016, Mr. President? Let it be **YOUR LEGACY** alone! A stroke of your pen could seal the deal. Leave Fast & Furious, IRS targeting, Benghazi, VA scandals, Unaffordable Health Care, a twenty trillion dollar debt, a weak economy and crushing unemployment woes behind you in the dust. **They can all become fast-faded memories.**

As is the case with tobacco and alcohol, please remove marijuana entirely from the Drug Schedules. At the very least reschedule marijuana to Schedule III or higher. You could do either by Executive Order! Decriminalize possession and use. <u>Allow the states to decide what their citizens demand</u>. Your legacy will be assured!

Legal marijuana can be a *trillion dollar <u>TAXABLE</u> INDUSTRY*, far surpassing alcohol, conventional tobacco and rivaling Big Pharma and Big Oil.

The savings throughout the legal system, courts, police and incarceration costs, together with the huge new tax revenue, would boost the economy, reduce the National Debt, and create many millions of new jobs. The plus side of the economic equation is *enormous*!

The stigma attached to marijuana busts and the resulting devastation of life-ruining conviction records, sadly **<u>disproportionately among inner city black youths</u>**, all can disappear in a flash. Mr. President, your legacy as a liberator of all oppressed minority classes will be remembered much as Abraham Lincoln and Martin Luther King are remembered.

Have we as a Nation learned nothing from the horrors of the thirteen-year alcohol Prohibition Era? To date apparently so. Compared to deadly alcohol consumption, which has been 100% legal since late in 1933, endless studies have shown that marijuana's potential for harm is non-existent.

Have we as a Nation learned nothing from the hundreds of thousands of American deaths attributed annually to smoking tobacco? To date, apparently we have learned very little.

It is morally corrupt to NOT arrest those who sell and use alcohol and tobacco, while labeling as criminals those who sell and use the far less harmful natural healing herb marijuana.

Have you forgotten our PTSD afflicted veterans, over twenty of whom commit suicide every day? What about the tens of thousands of black kids whose lives have been ruined by convictions and incarcerations for minor marijuana offenses? These situations can be permanently erased by a simple stroke of your mighty pen.

Mr. President, hear the plea of the people! Decriminalize, un-schedule or reschedule marijuana to Schedule III. Make it happen, the sooner the better. If you can change our public bathroom laws you can certainly do this. Don't allow some future President to take the credit and glory for something that **you** could do **NOW**!

Your golden legacy can be eternal!

GOD bless you sir, and GOD bless America.

J. Burton Anderson, Lions Pride Publishing

www.ingramcontent.com/pod-product-compliance
Lightning Source LLC
Chambersburg PA
CBHW062154270326
41930CB00009B/1534